How to Surviv
Psychotherapis.

HOW TO SURVIVE AS A PSYCHOTHERAPIST

Nina Coltart

sheldon **PRESS**

First published in Great Britain 1993
Sheldon Press, Marylebone Road, London NW1 4DU

British Library Cataloguing in Publication Data
A catalogue record for this book is available from the British
Library
ISBN 0–85969–665–0

5 7 9 10 8 6 4

Typeset by Inforum, Rowlands Castle, Hants
Printed and bound by Antony Rowe Ltd, Eastbourne

| *Contents*

For Agi Bene

Acknowledgements

From time to time in this book, I refer to 'Slouching Towards Bethlehem', which was my first paper. I would like to thank my friend, Gregorio Kohon, psychoanalyst and editor of *The British School of Psychoanalysis; The Independent Tradition* who included it in that book, and encouraged me to go on writing.

I acknowledge with gratitude the help of the following: Judith Longman, editorial director, Sheldon Press, who had the original idea for the book and invited me to write it; David Black, series consultant and also a psychoanalyst, who was the perfect middleman and helped me with planning the book; Ruth Levitt, who gave me constructive criticism throughout, and compiled the index; and finally, my old friend, Isabel Vincent, who not only accurately read my handwritten manuscript, but also skilfully edited it as she put it on the word processor. Finally, I would like to thank Christopher Bollas, who has discussed my writing with me, and encouraged me to continue.

Nina E.C. Coltart
September 1992

Introduction

The concept of survival became specialized as a result of the Second World War. All reasonably educated adults in the English-speaking world accept that the special meaning relates to the people who managed to live through the experience of Nazi Germany, and the concentration camps – predominantly Jews. It seems almost impertinent for an ordinary non-Jewish psychotherapist like me to use the term 'survival'. When we think of some of the long-drawn-out, quiet suffering of many Jewish survivors, and, as has been more recently realized, of their children and relatives, we are thinking of survival in its rawest, bleakest sense: that of simply continuing to live in this world, often irremediably scarred, helplessly exerting pathological influences on succeeding generations.

I think it is legitimate, however, to salvage the idea of survival to express something more light-hearted – a positive experience with much that is happy and creative in it. This is the meaning I want to give to the notion of 'surviving as a psychotherapist'. A teeth-gritting, desperate struggle against ferocious odds would imply a gross distortion of the whole idea of being a therapist. Unless the term can be used in a truly positive way, there would be little to be said for it. At the heart of the matter lies the idea of enjoyment: enjoyment of the experience which is being survived, and enjoyment of the ways in which it enriches the whole of the life of the survivor, whether working or relaxing, or simply being oneself.

1
Survival-with-Enjoyment

The working life of a full-time analytical psychotherapist is emotionally and psychologically a tough one, and it is this quality of toughness, with difficulties to be met and managed and overcome, which justifies the idea of survival. There is no particular merit in living through a day when the job to be done offers no challenge. Survival-with-enjoyment of necessity implies certain problems encountered and solved; hardships which require endurance and ingenuity and the deployment of energy, and which also bring in their train a particular sort of satisfaction as they begin to yield and become things of the past.

These are not enormous, primitive hardships such as hunger and cold, and again one feels the need to defend the use of language. But if we accept that the structure of our particular context – psychotherapy – is nevertheless bound to contain its own particular sorts of difficulty, then it is legitimate to say that, relative to the ease and enjoyment which is possible in enjoyable survival, problems can seem insuperable at times, and psychic hardships real, not an exaggerated use of language.

What are the problems in broad outline? Within this structure, which has an undeniable sophistication about it, the problems are loneliness of a certain sort, and the emotional strains of continually and voluntarily offering oneself to the inner suffering of other people in the hope – or faith – that there is something in the way this self-exposure is offered which may be of therapeutic aid to the other person.

High-class problems, they have been called; invisible to the passing glance of the general public; ludicrous even to think of complaining. And on the whole, we are not complaining. Whatever the content of a period of severe anxiety, or complete bafflement, or feeling hopelessly inadequate in the face of another person's massive unhappiness, we do know that we have *chosen* to be where we are. I think most of us would be extremely careful to restrict our grumbling or complaining to the sort of audience – most likely of peers or colleagues, or the family – who would either understand, or be inclined to take our word that to us our difficulties are very real.

What we seek, with justified hope, is survival-with-enjoyment. Being aware that the job itself can be a source of rich satisfactions, our focus of interest is not where to put our complaining, but how to survive with maximum happiness. For this, a rough map of some of the problems, an approximate geography of the 'danger areas', and some news from a thus-far-survivor-with-enjoyment come in handy both to those setting out on the journey, and those who are somewhere on the same journey.

I realized when I began to reflect on this subject that to write authentically about enjoyable survival I have to be somewhat more autobiographical than I had at first anticipated. This is not, after all, a simple 'How to . . .' handbook. If I were just to list a number of things which might assist you it would in no time become unbearably pedantic, or priggish, or counter-productively tiresome. Probably all three; and certainly inauthentic. How do I know these things, anyway? And who do I think I am, telling you how to be?

Surviving the first stage, that is, the training – which may cover anything up to five years or so – is a very different matter to surviving the later stages. Another way of saying this is that Getting There is a profoundly different matter from Being There. Probably it would be true to say that the early years of the second stage, Being There, are the hardest of the lot, and need the most detailed mapping. By comparison, Getting There is a doddle; smooth trekking, in gentle, wooded foothills, compared with some of the bleak (self-)exposed hard climbing of the next bit. And yet it may not feel like that at the time, and it is often only in retrospect that the young – or perhaps I should say, recently qualified – psychotherapist realizes that the difference is not just one of degree, but of entering a different dimension altogether.

The concept of 'young' has to be used with care; there are no other professions I can call to mind in which the newly qualified practitioner is likely to be as old as most of us are. In the world of academia, becoming a professor may be a relatively new experience and present new challenges to one who was, until that point, an ordinary member of a university department; but it is not qualitatively different in any major way. Newly qualified therapists are likely to be in their thirties, although they seem to be getting older now, and are often well into their forties.

What makes the first stage so different from all the rest? It is the nature of the training itself: the careful, complex structure, with its many well-defined constituents, surrounds the student in a therapy organization like a dedicated mother. It is the movement out of the training and into qualified practice that represents the great divide. In some cases, this closely supportive structure peels away slowly, or is abandoned by the ex-student in carefully planned stages; but often it falls away quite suddenly and completely, and one is where one has consciously longed to be – out on one's own. The subjective paradox of emerging, naked and inexperienced, from the training, while to all intents and purposes appearing to the world as before, a confident, responsible, middle-aged adult, can be one of the dangerous areas of hardship on the journey.

It has to be understood – and this is a feature which is strange to the lay public – that a student who is training to be a dynamic psychotherapist or a psychoanalyst is not the same kind of creature as is a student in any other context. For one thing, with us a student is always a postgraduate, whose normal student years were spent acquiring qualifications in medicine, psychology, social work, anthropology, and occasionally more outlying subjects.

The label 'student' – with its implications of lack of knowledge, power, and seniority – grates sourly on some people, who resent it throughout the training. Others find it refreshing to be in the position of learner again, expected to receive, not to give, and they relish the freedom from authoritative responsibility in at least this one section of their lives. I think this relishing response is an aid to survival; it should be possible to acquire it even if one's more characteristic inclination is to kick against it. One has, after all, elected to do this late training and, perhaps because there is a tendency to over-protection throughout the course, it should not be impossible to learn to sit back and enjoy it.

Most students are in full- or part-time employment, and have to fit the training round that as best they may. Although several psychotherapy societies are generous with loans and grants, they do not cover the training, and many students do not receive them. The training is extremely demanding of both money and time, which can be a source of aggravation unless it is firmly kept in mind that one is doing it by choice, and the economical path, emotionally speaking, is to extract as much pleasure from it as possible.

For some, the demands on time are more serious even than the financial ones. One has to be in either full analysis or an analytical therapy of some intensity, which is crucially the heart of the training. Two or three evenings a week are given over completely to attending lectures and seminars. The last two years of the full training also have to include several more unpaid hours, devoted to seeing one's training patients for a full psychotherapy, together with regular weekly sessions with a different supervisor for each case.

Since most training therapists, understandably, see their own patients (the trainees) in normal working hours, this means that roughly a minimum of twelve to seventeen hours in a working week is devoted, unpaid, to the training requirements. I say 'a minimum' because many students spend several more hours each working day journeying to and from sessions in heavy traffic. If one adds to the total of, say, many hours of daily appointments, including one's own therapy, and travelling, the ten or so evening hours of seminar work, it will readily be calculated that almost a full working week is given over to the latter part of the training, which may extend to well over two years if the student is not considered ready for qualification.

The demands of the training for analytical psychotherapists are slightly less than those required to become a full classical psycho-analyst, but are rigorous enough. Many of their students may elect to be in full analysis (i.e., five times a week) themselves, but the requirement, both for themselves and for their training patients, are for three-times-a-week attendance. Is it any wonder that 'survival', in its barest sense, comes to seem the precisely appropriate term for the student approaching the longed-for goal of getting out of the training and into – back into – independent life?

For the student who is married and trying to participate as fully as possible in the upbringing of a young family there are serious drawbacks; it seems to me that one of the reasons for a steady fall in the recruitment of really suitable applicants is ascribable solely to this. Senior trainers are sometimes accused of losing touch with the real world, and on occasion there seems to be sound justification for this suspicion. Long, serious discussions about the reasons why more thirty-year-old doctors do not apply to train often omit the horror of the prospect of giving up hours and hours of one's middle-life, when the children are growing up and professional work is anyway demanding enough.

There is a slight tendency among some elderly, single psycho-analysts (a group I am wary of, as I shall soon belong to it) to behave and speak as if a sufficient devotion to 'analysis' in the potential student will iron out all the problems in his/her way. This is anachronistic, pseudo-idealistic rubbish. A vocation may be strong, but the trainings are tougher than they were, and the logistical problems have a dreadful reality. Students often look, and are, completely exhausted as the breaks between training terms approach. Some marriages do not survive personal psychotherapy or analysis, and some of the students' children become disturbed.

There is also a tendency among a certain type of senior psychotherapist (overlapping with the group above) to suggest that both the spouses and the children should themselves undertake therapy, or even analysis, as if it were the sovereign remedy for all these ills. To my mind this again supports the lay view that we are alienated from everyday life. A massive family disturbance which is brought about by the demands of training that are laid on a husband and father/wife and mother, is not likely to be solved, or even helped, by further outlay of family resources in terms of time and money.

That survival-with-enjoyment can be a real problem is, I hope, clearer by now, although it can be achieved by the exercise of considerable ingenuity – and a strong vocational drive underlying the original choice. However, the distinct tendency to idealize 'psychoanalysis' and all that has grown from it is not helped towards dissolution by some of the attitudes of the student's trainers.

It may well be that this tendency to idealize analysis and its powers is both fostered by certain analysts and therapists during the training course, and necessary to the student to enable him/her to endure the taxing requirements. It is noticeable that the idealization begins to shrink, and eventually disappear – and that it should is right and desirable – fairly soon after the student qualifies (see Chapter 6). This suggests there are strong unconscious influences keeping it alive before qualification. The idealization goes hand-in-hand with the infantilizing effect of the training, which tends to be fostered by the very fact of being a student, and which the student may find it hard to escape even if he/she observes that it is occurring. All students are in their own psychotherapies, and there is no question that this exerts a regressive pull on even the most stable character. And of course, the most gifted students are not by any means always stable characters. That a 'normal' person is unlikely to be a gifted therapist is almost an *idée reçue* in our strange world.

I have used the word 'vocation' more than once, and I use it in spite of the fact that it arises from another context altogether – that of the religious aspirant. It is over-pedantic to insist that the word derives from a Latin root, *vocare*, 'to call' which implies there is a Caller. Candidates for our trainings are unlikely to be religious believers, at least in any theocentric religion, and by using the idea of vocation, I am referring to a profound emotional and intellectual conviction that one is pursuing a goal that is absolutely right for oneself – not to any religious notion that one is being 'called', for example, by God. It is important to make this clear; more than once I have found myself at cross-purposes with a 'believer' when using the word without explanation.

I believe that the strong sense of rightness for oneself of this particular path in life not only can justifiably be called a vocation, but also that it is this very vocational quality which is the source of the deepest and most sustained experience of survival-with-enjoyment. One will need to withstand a great deal of hardship in the pursuit of a vocation – indeed, the kind of patient endurance required is one of the recognized ways in which a vocation is tested. I am only enabled to tackle the subject of this book because I am absolutely sure, and have been for many years, that I am a round peg in a round hole; I had an unwavering sense of what I recognized as 'vocation' from the earliest days.

What I have referred to as the infantilizing effect of the training is linked to just how much there is to learn, especially when one is extremely ignorant of the whole field, as I certainly was when I began. For one thing, there is by now a vast literature, which increases almost week by week as a result of steady streams of new papers in the multiplicity of journals. Probably most therapists settle for selective reading from a regular subscription to not more than three or four journals at the most; any more would rapidly become persecutory. It must be clear from what I said earlier, that one's spare time is at a minimum during the student years, and one has only to do a few weeks of teaching, after qualification, especially of a theoretical subject, to realize that carefully prepared reading lists for the students should also be kept to a minimum. As bibliographies to be filed for future reference, lengthy reading lists may have their value; but any lecturer or seminar leader who seriously anticipates the students will have read them as current preparation is in for a disappointment. Of recent years I have confined myself to teaching Technique to final-year students – which is when they are becoming most keenly aware of needing some help with this subject – and I ask only that they prepare Freud's five or six papers on Technique (1912–14). This is partly

because they are wonderful papers, fresh and cogent and of immediate value, and partly because I believe that if during their training all students can read as much Freud as possible, they have at
least started to incorporate the foundation on which all the rest of
the massive literature is based.

The most striking change after qualification is the disappearance
of all the detailed care and attention which is lavished on students.
Many do not anticipate just how great their loss will be, and it is
only the contrast which brings it home to them. Personal therapy
often continues for some years after qualification, and it is the
ending of that which is the deepest bereavement; while it continues, the loss of other forms of personal care may well be muted.
Nevertheless, it is noticeable.

Each student is allocated a progress adviser throughout the
training. This person, a training analyst or senior training therapist, functions rather as a moral tutor does at Oxbridge – a reliable
senior person to whom the student can turn with any problems
that may occur, and which are not appropriately handled, in a
practical sense, in the personal analytical therapy. Many students
make quite extensive use of their progress advisers, and this relationship ceases on qualification.

Supervisors vary in their styles of managing the training case
work. Some may continue to see the ex-student for a while; others, of whom I am one, make it clear that supervision comes to an
end very shortly after qualification. My own reason for this is that
I consider that, unless the work is very shaky, the sooner the
newly qualified therapist is out on his/her own, the better.
Therapy is essentially a craft where self-reliance is the order of the
day. The sooner these middle-aged adults emerge from the co-
cooning of the training, the sooner they will begin to realize this.

The fullest realization comes with the end of their own personal
analyses or therapies. Surviving this chain of losses can be the
hardest passage in all one's life as a therapist; an enormous quantity of emotional investment now has to be slowly withdrawn and
redeployed. The bereavement is very real, following the severance
of a relationship which often has been among the most important
of one's life.

Much has been written about termination, though nothing
which surpasses Freud's great, grim paper of 1937 'Analysis Terminable and Interminable'.[1] I do not propose to examine the literature here, but one thing needs to be stated in this context, if only
because, rather oddly, it is rarely referred to directly. I wonder

whether we do not collectively turn a blind eye to the extra-ordinary paradox of the intensely artificial nature of this key rela-tionship, which nevertheless can only thrive and 'work' if both participants, from their different standpoints, enter into it in an authentic way. All the emotions experienced in analytical therapy are real; the extending of one's psychic boundaries through work and insight is real; the intensity and the (illusory) power of the transference are real. Yet the relationship – unique as it is throughout – has to be terminated in a uniquely arbitrary way. Whatever may be said – and it is, at length – about 'criteria for termination', being 'ready to end', and so on, the fact of termina-tion is completely artificial. In saying this, I am most certainly not advocating that the relationship should be continued, or that grad-ual socialization should replace the uniquely asymmetrical thera-peutic intensity. On the contrary, I adhere strictly to the belief that the end should be as absolute as possible, for the sake of the patient's freedom from me. I only wish to underline the odd fact of the arbitrary and long-anticipated nature of this often severe loss, which is inherent in the whole process.

During the termination phase of any analysis or long psycho-therapy, it is generally accepted that there may appear not only symptom recurrence in brief, condensed forms, but also that pre-vious experiences of separation in the patient's life may be emo-tionally recalled, with the opportunity of working through them in a deeper, more detailed way than was possible at the time. However, one of the psychic hardships to which I referred may confront the emerging student (patient) at this stage. Indeed, it is this one in particular which constitutes the change from one di-mension of experience to another.

It is perfectly possible to bring about changes in the ego by means of dynamic therapy such that it is forever stronger, more resilient, more able to cope with, among other things, severe sepa-ration pain. But beyond a certain point, it is not possible to antici-pate (in order to protect against) the actual experience of loss. Psychotherapy may well prepare the ground for a more adequate capacity to mourn, but, paradoxically, because the ego can allow for a more flexible range of emotions, the mourning which truth and health require may be more painful than it would have been previously. Freud, and many writers since his time, always insisted that analysis, and all therapy deriving from it, is not designed to shield one from reality – only to make it both richer and more manageable. There used to be an advertising slogan which stated:

'There is no substitute for wool'. When it comes to ending this kind of therapy, there is, however careful the foregoing termination work has been, no substitute for ending. It is precisely the sufferings caused by ending, the pain of bereavement, even symptoms, which most fully test the value of the therapy itself, since by definition they are the first sufferings for several years which one is unable to take into the 'comforting container' as one has become so accustomed to doing.

Someone like myself, with a long-past experience of double parental loss at a vulnerable stage in life (early adolescence) may be impelled to rework much of the ground which of course received considerable attention during my analysis. I found it at times difficult to discriminate between sadness which was brought forward from the past, and the sadness truly attaching to the mourning for my own analysis. Perhaps it did not matter; the necessary inner working got done eventually, and gratitude for what one had received, particularly the capacity for ongoing self-analysis, was a strong contribution to survival at that time. The detached, observing self could study, in finer detail than had ever been possible before, the different stages of mourning as they were reached, worked through, and left behind. It was the testing of this enhanced capacity for a real interest in the emotional progress in oneself that made for a new sort of survival. One of the features which aroused my strongest interest was an appreciation of the role played by identification with the lost person in healthy mourning; I realized as never before the degree to which identifications with both my parents, a doctor-father and a psychologically minded mother, had played a major role in what I had naïvely thought were my own independent choices of profession and lifestyle. And this realization came about, of course, through the identification with my own analyst, which is, partly, what self-analysis is.

Do not, by the way, think that the actual event of qualification transforms the student into 'an analyst' or 'a therapist' overnight. He or she will have learned a great deal quite fast during the training, and, especially if they have already established a practice, will be just beginning to gain experience of the application of their learning to the problems which confront them. But the slow development of a skilful, flexible technique, the constant new angles on what is intellectually known, and the gradual reduction of anxiety all take a long time. On the day I qualified, I was cock-a-hoop, and probably thoroughly over-sanguine. My analyst said,

'Yes, that's good that the training is behind you. Now it will take another ten years for you to become an analyst.' I was somewhat deflated, but in retrospect I know she was right.

Try to keep some space in your mind free from the very prevalent 'beginner's anxiety'. It does gradually fade away, as you slowly master and internalize what is to be truly yours; and as your learning sinks down into the reservoirs of the unconscious, you will move more freely in each session, and become steadily more confident.

It may well be that many newly qualified therapists, leaving behind their own personal psychotherapy, do not have an earlier life-event which both enriches and makes more painful this particular stage; but I know that some do, and I also know that most do need to learn at this point to mourn, and that this experience strengthens them for the future. One grows through this time, painfully and yet with a deep sense of satisfaction. The great life-event of one's own therapy and the ending of it settle gradually into their rightful place in one's mind. With perhaps a little help from luck, and with a real and enjoyable base for building one's new professional identity, one embarks on the next stage of the journey.

2
Psychoanalysis vs. Psychotherapy?

In the course of the large number of consultations I have done during the last twenty-five years, I am often asked, 'What is the difference between psychoanalysis and psychotherapy?' The rather oddly placed question mark in the title of this chapter appeared because I have never been able to formulate a clear, concise answer to this question. I wish I could. Consultations would flow on more easily if I could produce a brief, explanatory paragraph which satisfied the intelligent questioner.

What I usually say, though not at all satisfactory to me, does address some of the more practical points which are relevant, and which are in the mind of the patient, jostling with imaginative anxiety about whatever I am currently prescribing. It is something along the lines of, 'They both try to explore the hidden layers of the mind, which are probably contributing to your problems at the moment; they both rely on your doing a lot of the work, and learning to speak freely about whatever you are thinking then and there. Analysis is a bigger commitment; the patient needs to have sessions very frequently – four or five times a week – because the intensity and continuity are so valuable. Psychotherapy requires only once to three times a week sessions.' Really, all I have done is use frequency of sessions as my main differentiating factor, other-wise I have in fact described similarity.

As the title of this book indicates, I am not a full-time, five-times-a-week-or-nothing psychoanalyst. Insofar as there are dif-ferences between 'doing psychoanalysis' and 'doing psycho-therapy', my first love has always been psychotherapy. Before I explain this, let us have a brief overview of the history of tradi-tional, mainstream psychoanalysis, and the way in which some of the breakaway movements have set up the patterns, and some-times the foundations, of the various practices which have collec-tively become known as psychotherapy.

Freud said he was not particularly interested in treating ill people; what he valued about psychoanalysis was that it provided an inves-tigative technique for exploring the workings of the human psyche. It is difficult for us to imagine now how unbelievably innovative it was that, for this purpose, Freud introduced the practice of seeing people five, or even six, times a week. Not only that, but he got them to lie on the couch, behind which he would sit. While this is now one of the traditional features of psychoanalysis, and many are the theories which have accumulated round this radical piece of technique, they all stand on the simple, fundamental fact that Freud hated being stared at for so many hours a week. Freud of course rationalized this innovation at once, saying here and there in his writings that both patient and analyst could 'free associate' more easily in this position, and the analyst could use his only instrument, himself – his reactions and his unconscious – to tune in to that of the patient without the obstacle of visual information.

As it happened, those who learned Freud's method brought more enthusiasm than he did to the idea of using the technique thera-peutically, because for most of us his great discovery was that people with psychological symptoms seemed to benefit from it.

Since the early part of the century, there have been only small numbers of people who have used the full Freudian technique of psychoanalysis. Nevertheless, it is upon psychoanalysis that most forms of dynamic psychotherapy are based, however far removed they may be, and however much people who believe, or pretend, that they have invented them, may argue their original merits.

There were a number of such offshoots already in the first years of the 'psychoanalytical movement', as it was known. Prominent among them was Jung, whose thought and methods differ exten-sively from Freud's. In the field of dynamic therapy, his system is still the biggest rival to Freud's, in this sense perpetuating the rivalrous enmity which grew up between the two men. Jung wrote about his theoretical differences with the analyst who had once been his revered teacher; Freud in turn looked upon Jung for a while as his heir apparent.

Since these differences have grown and crystallized over the years, the theory, technique, and language of analytical psychol-ogy, as it has become known, contrast markedly with all work based on that of Freud. For example, there is less importance attached to the two great well-springs of Freudian theory, sex and aggression; Freud's structural theory of the mind, worked out in the 1920s, is abandoned, and Jung, who believed himself to have mystical experiences, emphasized the whole spiritual dimension, unlike Freudian reductionist technique, which virtually ignores it as a psychological entity.

A long-term result of this is that many people who are religiously observant and value their spirituality turn naturally to Jungians when looking for analytic help; a secondary result of *that* is that analysts and therapists in the Freudian tradition do not have experience of dynamic work with religious people sufficient to broaden their views intelligently from the dismissive prejudices which Freud himself undoubtedly harboured.

Others who embarked on new versions of psychoanalysis, often as the result of personal quarrels with Freud – a patriarch who brooked little criticism, and was easily hurt by disloyalty – either gained few adherents and their deaths saw the end of their ventures, or else emphasized a particular aspect of Freud's enormous range of new ideas, and used it in such a way that their names live on today, attached to various rather specialized schools of analytic thought.

Among those who did not start a tradition were Otto Rank, whose thinking was already potentially present in the main body of post-Freudian thought, and Victor Tausk, whose 'original views' turned out to be the onset of psychosis. Rank developed a preoccupation with the importance of what he saw as the trauma of birth, and tended to trace everything back to that; his influence can be seen today in variations such as primal scream therapy, which originated in the United States and became somewhat popular about twenty years ago. Even R.D. Laing, probably the most famous, least stereotyped, psychoanalyst our modern Freudian tradition has produced, was for a while interested in trying to take people back to the very beginnings of their individual lives.

Early psychoanalysts whose eponymous therapies still flourish among certain sections of society include, besides Jung, Alfred Adler and Wilhelm Reich. Adler emphasized the will to power, based on what he thought of as 'organ inferiority', supposedly discoverable in a remarkable number of people. Reich, though in the opinion of many seriously mad for the latter part of his life, had a charisma with which he imbued his strange ideas about transformation and the Orgone Box, and which to this day attracts people with sexual problems. A recent 'breakaway' analyst was Jacques Lacan in France, who has a large following among intellectuals, especially neuro-psycho-linguistics specialists, as well as the more general world of academia. Lacan's technical fireworks contrast more sharply with staid old psychoanalysis than do his main central theoretical ideas.

Let us move on from this brief sketch of some of the outgrowths from psychoanalysis and try to define what it is that we all – psychoanalysts and psychotherapists from any and all analytic training schools – hold in common. I think I can assume the following. First, we all accept the existence, in all people, of an unconscious mental life which is alive, active, and often full of conflicts, and which constantly influences our thinking and behaviour. Second, our therapeutic work is directed towards exploring and revealing the contents and structure of the unconscious, with a view to the person becoming the master, rather than the slave, of its power. Third, in our work as interpreters of the unconscious, as frequently and as creatively as we can, we use our observations of the conscious and unconscious transference feelings of the patient towards us, and the conscious and unconscious (by self-analysis) counter-transferences – i.e., all the information made available to us by our total reactions to the patient.

Now I will try to explain why psychotherapy has always been my first love. It will not necessarily coincide with other people's views, but for the purposes of this book it gives my working definition of therapy, and an idea of the distinctions I make between therapy and analysis.

In therapy, I am referring to patients who come at the most three times a week, usually twice, sometimes once. The majority of them would be sitting up in a chair, facing me, as I prefer more direct interaction. I would use the transference, to make transference interpretations, as often as I could, but I would not anticipate that this would take up the greater part of the work as I would expect it to if I were doing full analysis (four or five times a week, patients on the couch).

In most sessions I would expect to engage in dialogue on many levels, and included in that dialogue would be much material that, strictly speaking, is extra-transference, but of current or past importance to the patient. Whatever bits of technique I am using at that moment, I would at all times endeavour to listen past the overtly conscious content, and to indicate to the patient that I am doing so. I would make plenty of allowance for the fact that I have an expressive face, and would not attempt to maintain a dead-pan expression. I would allow freer rein to my spontaneity, and would not be afraid of expressing more emotion, of whatever kind, than I would if engaged on a full analysis. I would expect jokes and laughing to be part of what happens in some sessions unless the material strictly indicates otherwise. I would, at times, express an opinion on matters of fact which might conceivably affect the patient's subsequent behaviour – which I would then expect to be discussed. In short, whatever, 'engaging with the patient' in the fullest possible way means to me would be my aim when 'doing psychotherapy'.

I do not suppose for a moment that there will be instant agreement with all the above points, but that, among psychotherapists, agreement with some, or with the overall picture, would seem likely. Of course, objections to any point that I have made arise naturally, whether it is 'therapy' or 'analysis' which is under discussion. For one thing, all analysis is therapy, but not all therapy is analytic, in the broadest meanings of the terms. For another, individuals provide exceptions simply through the infinite vagaries of being human. One elderly man sat up throughout a long and complex classical analysis.[1] Another man, in his forties, always refused to come more than once a week, yet insisted on lying on the couch. He produced material in such a way that I could never have abandoned constant transference interpretation even if I had wanted to. He called his treatment – quite properly in my view – 'my analysis'.

This strongly suggests that my definition of 'analysis' has a lot to do with my type of regular response to the patient, and not so much to do with the frequency of sessions; this makes good sense to me. We all encounter, at times, the sort of patient who simply *makes one do analysis*, pulls it out of one. Such patients are very enjoyable to work with, and completely meet my criteria for psychological-mindedness (see Chapter 6).[2] In contrast, I recall another man, a deeply neurotic and rather typical philosopher, who always wanted to watch me, though he lay on the couch. So I sat, rather uncomfortably at first, in what was for me a peculiar position (strict practitioners will say I should have analyzed his wish rather than complying with it; had he been psychologically-minded, I would have done so). Each day I had to drag my chair to a place near the end of the couch, and face him. He was painfully clever, like many academic intellectuals I have met; and this bizarre twosome engaged in the most humdrum conversations every day, dominated largely by his need to list obsessionally practically everything he had done since he last saw me. However I tried to interpret this litany, I made not the slightest impact. He would wait until I had delivered myself of some (to me) increasingly boring interpretation, nod cordially, and say in a considered, heavy way, 'I see – yes, that's most interesting', and continue as before. I could not call that a psychoanalysis unless I were devoted only to form; content and technique were more like nursery-school supervision.

I do not mean to convey by any invidious sort of comparison process that I do not enjoy doing psychoanalysis. I do, very much; but I do think it is *easier* than what I am defining as psychotherapy. Dynamic psychotherapy seems to me to keep one at full stretch all the time; although people are capable of surprising one indefinitely, and unexpected flashes of thought and insight certainly arise during the course of an analysis, the very classicism of the container means there is less scope for adventures of the spirit. However subtle and flexible one's technique becomes over the years, there are certain sorts of determined types of response to many situations. Especially in a training analysis, there are great blocks of theory which, if they come up, have to be worked on.

Having said that, I feel the need to add that I do not think a training analysis should be fundamentally different from any other. As I said earlier, many analytic students – and psychotherapy students having an analytic training therapy – are ill, disturbed, gifted people; if they have not needed their training analysis as a therapeutic experience for themselves, they are unlikely to be as sensitive and empathic with other psychologically disturbed people. Patients who have rather unusual forms of disease, such as highly specialized perverts, sometimes say, 'I don't see how you can understand what I'm talking about. I'm quite sure you've never known anything like this yourself.' Of course, if this person is a shoe fetishist or likes being tied up in chains and beaten, this is most likely to be correct. But, having undergone the analysis of some discomforting areas of ourselves – and bearing in mind that many of Freud's early discoveries, and therefore his writings, were via contact with perversions – we do know something, enough, we hope, of the analytic method to which psychopathology yields to be able to unravel and enlighten, if not always to change.

Whichever way I turn on this subject, there is the possibility of objection being raised. All the arguments can be supported. And there have been periods in carrying out psychoanalysis that have been among the most difficult I have ever encountered, and I'm sure that most colleagues with mixed practices could say the same.

There is a huge psychic advantage in four- or five-times weekly analysis: however tricky and tense the point at which a session has to stop, at least the patient is returning on the morrow to take it up again. The analyst will not lose touch with the acutely sensitive area, and the patient will not have to contain his anxiety or misery for too long alone. On the other hand, there is a lot to be said for a rest period. Time, however short – say, a week – does have healing properties as well as disadvantages. One of the problematic features of some analytic difficulties lies, *for the therapist*, in the very fact that there is only twenty-four hours' respite before one has to plunge into the maelstrom again. This may not allow enough time for really thorough unconscious processing, although a night's sleep can sometimes achieve a surprising amount of work.

One of the most refreshing and enjoyable things about getting older is that the anxiety from which I used to suffer a great deal while working has completely disappeared. It may disappoint my patients and ex-patients to learn that I now rarely think about them between sessions, trusting to my unconscious to do the necessary work; it is because that trust is repaid over and over again that anxiety has gone. If I find I am thinking about a patient, then I know there is a real cause for concern; it is on such an occasion that a good night's sleep – particularly if a revealing dream is recalled – can provide the space and relaxation for condensed, and often enlightening, work.

A very positive aspect is precisely that the luxurious frequency of a four- or five-times-a-week treatment means that one can grapple with a problem at close quarters. Quite apart from the intrinsically therapeutic effect of simply doing it, the learning potential for both therapist and patient of such microscopically detailed work is immense.

One cannot *un*learn, or not know, some tiny bit of theory which has come to life before one's very eyes in the moment-to-moment exploration of a deep, intensive session. The perversions provide excellent opportunities for such work: the dramatic and relentlessly repetitive nature of perverse symptomatology lays out the template of early psychosexual development so clearly that it provides a better learning experience than any amount of reading or number of good seminars. There is also a degree of adaptiveness to transference work in such patients, which, together with the striking pathology, makes them extraordinarily instructive.

This does not mean, unfortunately, that the outcome is always good; on the whole it is not, and it is as well to be aware of this. It was a man with a complicated perversion who gave me almost my first taste of this, and who is often at the back of my mind when I urge students to treat a perverse patient if they possibly can. Radical change in psychic structure is anyway quite rare, and there is something determinedly fixated about most perversions, especially if a willing partner is found and the perverse fantasy is frequently acted out. However apparently responsive to detailed transference work the patient is, it is as if the fear of difference, and the stubborn, masochistic addictiveness to the selected sexual pattern render him inaccessible to change. This can be baffling to the still-idealistic young therapist, who expects good transference work, resulting in insight, to 'work'.

Wilfred Bion's invaluable piece of advice to all analytical therapists inevitably comes to mind. What he said – more than once, and by now it is so well known that the exact origin is forgotten – was that one should approach every session with every patient 'without memory and without desire'.[3] There is a danger that this piece of advice is now accepted as a truism, and that it is well known rather than well understood. I reach it in this context not only because I believe that understanding it is important, but because I think it is more applicable to a full analysis than to psychotherapy.

Students and young therapists tend not to accept Bion's statement as a truism, but to question it, saying, for example, 'How can you not have your memory?', and, 'Surely you have hopes for your patient?' Deeper reflection – and perhaps some reading of Bion – clarify it further. Bearing in mind that it is easier to sustain if one is seeing a patient five times a week, although one's memory is of course not erased but is ready and waiting to be drawn on at any moment, then ideally one should not embark on a session with expectations based on yesterday's work, or recent themes, or what one already knows of the patient's mind and its predictable patterns. Bion's view was that this sort of predictiveness has an influence which can obscure the complete openness of the therapist to receive anything that comes from the patient in free associations or in non-verbal signals. The implication is that one is ever ready to be surprised, and to begin to process all the bits of emerging material.

The advice that neither should one have 'desire' is harder to grasp, but Bion believed – and so do I – that by the use of the will, the therapist can work on himself, with the aim of *not* subtly imposing on the patient any specific hopes or wishes for him to 'get better'. While this seems contrary to the meaning of our role as would-be helpers and healers, it is a paradox rather than a contradiction. Insofar as we choose to operate in a branch of the healing profession, Bion does not mean that we should adopt an attitude which is alien to our main intention. I think he means that the danger lies in adopting *any* attitude: it is perfectly possible, within the moral boundaries of our work, to be almost infinitely flexible relative to each individual patient. If we 'desire' that he achieves an immediate goal – gets on better with his wife, becomes happier – our motivation may seem impeccable, but in fact we shall be imposing on him our own view of the situation, our own definitions of 'better' or 'happier'. In every session there has to be a genuine freedom from the dictates of our own memories of the patient, and from the subtle influences of our good-hearted wishes and hopes for him. There is a powerful prescription here for us, and if on inspection we observe that we – and therefore our patients – are not fully granted such freedom by us then there is work to be done, perhaps self-analytical, and certainly moral.

I have found it easier to fulfil Bion's dictum when seeing a patient very frequently, and also when he is psychologically-minded (see Chapter 6). With a patient who is coming once or twice a week, it can be important to use the memory, though never to allow desires to dominate our attitude. Themes which flow on fluently from day to day may suffer when there is an interruption of a week: the patient's resistances may take advantage of the lapse of time to sidestep a painful subject. Especially in a focal, or brief, treatment, such as the sixteen sessions of cognitive-analytic therapy, it is the job of the therapist to rescue the pair of them from dead ends or false trails.

The patient is genuinely in need of help, and it is up to us to exert ourselves and offer it. It is not appropriate, and it is not good therapy, to sit in lofty 'analytic' silence, and watch the whole enterprise foundering, secure in our narcissistic self-satisfaction that we are doing just what Bion suggested. Hence the importance to us of differentiating, *at least in our own minds*, the one, psychotherapy, from the other, psychoanalysis. Our view of *what* we are doing can profoundly influence *how* we do it.

Having outlined the shared, underlying principles of all dynamic therapy, and then discussed how analysis differs from therapy, I would like to bridge any sense of a gap by returning to the sorts of experience we may all have, whatever our chosen mode of training and working.

There have been occasional patients, relatively straightforward on first encounter, who gave me surprises when the therapy got going. Of course one could argue that in some way everybody is a sort of surprise. It is not just a tired old cliché to say that everyone is different; it is a repeated revelation. One would think that after thirty years I would know backwards and forwards and inside-out some types of person, and be able to predict a fair amount about them, beforehand and as a treatment unfolded. Up to a point there is some truth in this. But it would be a fatal mistake to start thinking like that; I cannot but imagine that one would half-consciously start imposing patterns on people, which is exactly what Bion was warning against. Not only would it detract from the constant, fresh interest which is such a living contribution to the survival of the therapist's own freshness of approach, but one would either be in for frequent rude shocks, or one would get into such deep muddy waters that communication would grind to a halt.

A conscious and careful preservation of one's *tabula rasa* capacities, turning a blank and receptive surface towards every patient in every session, is the best way of recruiting the services of one's own unconscious. One will only survive to the end, with at least some of one's early enthusiasm unclouded, if one can retain this capacity for surprise. As well, the patients may be able to surprise you repeatedly, but you must hope to surprise them, too. If a flash of understanding arises in the therapist, and can then be offered to the patient in a vivid, succinct way, the interpretation will stay with that patient long after the bulk of the work has sunk down into the silt of his mind. The capacity to grab something from a new angle, or to see past the immediate point to a meaning which will speak to the patient, is one to be grateful for. From the earliest days of practice, one has to nurture such innate gifts as one has for doing this uniquely odd job. To begin with, these gifts are only available in embryonic form, and need to grow in a particular atmosphere.

Whatever the style of the therapy, the atmosphere is in itself unique, and consists of a receptivity to every bit of information that a patient is conveying, from the beginning of every session; not just in what is said, but in the overall body language, tones of voice, tiny movements, minor appearances of symptoms, changes in muscular tension and in breathing, colour, gaze, hand gestures. It may be argued that a patient on the couch does not give one much opportunity for this; certainly one of the main reasons for my love of psychotherapy is the richness of information available when one can see the patient, and when the pace of the interchange is often faster. Nevertheless, one can glean a lot about couch patients when every sense is on the alert. For example, a patient who smells unpleasant, or who suddenly starts to smell one day, or even during a session, is saying something somatic, and – socially taboo though the subject is – we are obliged to make reference to it when most appropriate, and try to translate it. Valuable work can be achieved if one makes the effort to overcome one's conditioned reluctance to take up the matter by comment or interpretation.

The sharp, fleeting glance in the waiting room can be brimming with information. It was one of those rapid mental snapshots that gave me a private nickname for a patient, something which, arising spontaneously from one's own unconscious, can be richly descriptive. This particular patient, a small, slight, depressed woman whom I hardly knew at all, was sitting hunched over the fire in the low chair. 'Little Hedgehog', I thought to myself. And she was. This occurred in the second week of an analysis, so there had been hardly any opportunity for self-exposure by this woman, who was anyway painfully inhibited, and became a silent patient.[4] Later she became extremely prickly, spiky, resistant, almost literally rolling herself into a ball on the couch, with her face to the wall. But she was also a gambler, and a terrible risk-taker, as I discovered when she finally began to 'uncurl'.

It is not only therapists whose intuition throws up a nickname for a patient; it often happens the other way round, too, but we don't always get to know about it. One that I did hear cropped up most appositely from a patient of mine who had a great deal of money, but who was in some ways a typically anal character – mean, grudging, bullying and sadistic – which served as an armour protecting a rather gentle, timid, and loving person. One day I was trying to pierce this defensive armour by interpretation of quite a confronting, vivid type, using directly anal language. The patient resisted stubbornly at every turn. Nothing was willingly taken in, and very little was allowed out. The talk veered off in the direction of a conversation he had had with his wife the night before, an apparent change of subject. During that conversation he had been referring to me, and he said, 'I was telling her about that session when you said – only I don't call you Dr Coltart, I – ', and he stopped abruptly. 'No, I can't tell you what I call you behind your back', he added. 'Oh do', I said unceremoniously. He blushed and began to giggle, looking for all the world like a naughty schoolboy (he was sixty-two). 'Well—', (long pause) 'Old Fartarse', he said, and roared with laughter. It was an opportunity too good to miss. 'And *still* you don't like what I've just been saying', I said. He had to admit that it all made a lot of sense. I am a bit suspicious when I hear therapists talking about 'a breakthrough', as I think that rather dramatic word is a very unusual occurrence in our work. But this was as near as I have ever come to one, for that man, in that therapy.

In order to nurse along such gifts as one may have, whether it be analysis or therapy, one has to give oneself plenty of mental room in which to cultivate a spacious stillness of mind where insight and ideas can grow from one's relationship with the patient. And, at the same time as remaining modest and humble, and not stamping on the patient with cleverness and bits of theory one happens to have understood or retained, I think one must encourage a healthy, vigorous faith in one's own intuition, as exemplified in the spontaneous arising of nicknames and the seizing of opportunities to make contact.

The British, especially the middle classes with some pretensions to being well-educated, have been deeply conditioned not to be what is called conceited, or too 'pleased with themselves'. Although this may not be so strong or so detrimental to self-confidence as it was sixty or seventy years ago, it is still quite marked. But if we do not trust ourselves, and the power of our intentions and training and intuition, all combined, to have creative ideas about our patients, we are lost, and towards the end of our working lives we will not have survived as happily as we should. It is not conceited or stupidly over-confident, it is a sign of health and development, if, within the strict boundaries assimilated during our training, we can believe we are capable of having good ideas and insights, and say so, and use them. Only thus will we gradually shed the anxieties of early days in the practice, and work towards a freer, more enjoyable road to survival in our chosen therapeutic field.

3
Apparent Trivia

The title and contents of this chapter evolved out of a talk I gave many years ago to the staff of Ashburn Hall, a therapeutic community type of psychiatric hospital in Dunedin, New Zealand. I had not long reached the stage of feeling that my private practice was securely established, and I had realized that there are many details involved in setting it up and keeping it going that never quite seem to fit into any discussions in seminars during the training.

I have opened a discussion of this subject with many therapists in different parts of the world. The lively talk that ensues, and the eagerness with which students and therapists welcome thinking about the minutiae, which are nevertheless essentials, has led me to the belief that, while these do not exactly constitute the makings of an 'important paper', and since the net result of getting such 'trivia' right certainly contributes to the relaxed survival of the therapist, they are important enough to deserve a place somewhere.

I want to emphasize the word 'relaxed': for a therapist with a full-time private practice, the working day is going to be spent in what by most people's standards is an eccentrically low-key way. The therapist is going to sit for eight to ten hours a day in one of two chairs, in the same room. Patients will come and go, and for long periods of time the patient population will be unchanging, such is the length of the kind of therapy we offer. Does it not seem there is considerable value, therefore, in getting this working context right? What is right for one may well be wrong for another, in fine detail, but there are a number of things which demand our most scrupulous attention if we are going to be as relaxed as possible, in order to play our part, with our minds at rest, in the many difficult situations which people inevitably bring into our consulting rooms. Once that attention has been given to these details, most of them will become so much a constant part of our environment that we cease to think about them; and we can do that most comfortably if we get them right in the first place – for us. The attention lavished on them repays us a hundredfold – because they no longer matter.

There is no particular order to these trivia, though some are at the top of some hierarchy of importance, and some recur and demand renewed attention from time to time. First among the latter category must be the question: how does one get patients? It is no good setting up in a pleasing milieu if it remains empty: an environment, as a container, is designed to contain us-being-therapists, and we cannot be therapists if we have no patients.

Perhaps this is the place to include a brief look at the nomenclature itself. I have long observed, and it crops up more often today than it used to, a distinct division between those of us who refer to 'patients', and those who prefer to say 'clients'. The reason it crops up more frequently in recent years is, I think, that a form of treatment called 'counselling' has greatly increased in popularity. There are organizations which specifically undertake to train and produce counsellors; and counsellors tend to speak of 'clients'. Some 'alternative therapists' seem undecided and waver between the two; analysts and most dynamic therapists use 'patient'.

Anyone whose primary training was in medicine feels more at home with the word 'patient', and among these I count myself. In fact, I have a distinct aversion to the word 'client'. To me, a client is someone who is part of a transaction which is purely commercial, and which has nothing to do with the inner emotional life of the buyer. Hairdressers and banks have clients. I find it hard to understand the argument put forward by therapists who prefer to use 'clients': namely that people don't want to be designated as ill, or be seen to need therapeutic attention. Such people see the word 'patient' as stripping dignity (or what I have heard called 'person-hood'). I am inclined to think an oversensitivity is at work, probably in the purveyor of the counselling or therapy rather than the person on the receiving end. To me, 'patient' is an honourable old word, stemming from the Latin root, *patio*, 'I suffer'. People who come to us *are* suffering. It feels to me far more careful of their dignity if we allow for that, rather than trying to cloak their pain under some false notion that we are the vendors of something without emotional colouring, or that people are not really in sometimes desperate need, which we are trying to meet.

A dislike of the word 'patient' arises from a mistaken application of the concept of equality. It is, I believe, a paranoid anxiety to get upset about any notion of 'inequality' between therapist and patient. In human terms there is no question of inequality, but in professional terms, there *is* asymmetry. This is a useful and accurate way of looking at the therapeutic relationship: people would not ask for therapy, and be willing to pay for it and suffer for it if the therapist did not possess some knowledge and skills which the patient could locate elsewhere – say, among friends – for nothing. Money plays an important part in the transaction, of that there is no doubt, but this does not justify the notion of a 'client', as in an ordinary commercial exchange, since what is being purveyed has no equal in any other buying and selling relationship. It is of a different order.

Let us return to the question of finding patients. Although there is something unseemly in the idea of touting for custom, one cannot just sit back in one's chair and wait for a suffering world to beat a path to one's door. One has made a colossal outlay of time and money and emotional effort for many years in order to reach this point, and now, here it is: one is a therapist, ready to go, and one is probably in debt, and may have abandoned a paid job to make space for the practice, and here is the space, waiting to be filled.

Students are well advised to keep their ears open during the training for sources of referral. Some students may be noticed in clinical seminars by reason of being gifted, and seminar leaders may act on this and start to send them patients. Also there is usually a smallish number of senior analysts and therapists who are in contact with prospective patients, who see numbers of them in consultation, and need to make referrals. Of recent years I have been in the agreeable position of being able to refer a great many patients to a great many therapists, thus matching needs in ways which themselves require a particular sort of skill. I have always used the method of spotting promising students during clinical seminars. Therapists who are embarking on building up a practice should not be afraid to contact the people who do consultations, in order to introduce themselves and their needs, and to ask for help; they in turn may be able to fulfil the same role later in their lives. Shortly after I qualified, three senior analysts each referred an analytic patient to me; I never forgot those particular patients, who formed the cornerstone of the practice, and were of inestimable value to my confidence during a time of maximum anxiety.

I should add that patients may materialize from unlikely sources if one is, crudely speaking, opportunistic. One of my most appropriate referrals for analysis came through my dentist, and another from a venerable member of the clergy. Such people are often baffled as to where to turn if a friend is in need, and one is entirely justified in modestly suggesting oneself if one needs patients.

Now we come to the apparent trivia of one's practice, which may usefully be divided into two main sections: the setting, and the management of the practice.

The setting is the basically unchanging environment of one's working life. For desirable relaxation and forgetting about it for most of the time, it is essential that one is comfortable and happy in it, and that the details are right. The room is not a cell, and we are not condemned to it; it is a place in which we choose to live for much of the time, and I think it is perfectly permissible for it to reflect our personal choices. Of course, we shall have to handle comments, often critical, about these from patients as they begin to sense the freedom of expression which we encourage, and which is, indeed, the raw material of analytical therapy; we should not, however, be swayed in arranging our setting by any doubtful thoughts about what other people may or may not like.

A comfortable and well-sprung couch is necessary for all therapists whose style includes having patients lie down. Far more important for our own personal needs is a comfortable armchair, or two if some patients sit up. I cannot emphasize enough how essential a good chair is for sheer survival purposes. It is worth spending both time and money to ensure it is exactly right, and it is necessary to remind oneself, as the shop assistant starts shifting from foot to foot and glancing at his watch, that it may be necessary to sit in a chair for more than a minute or two, if this primary (I could almost say only) tool of our trade is to fit the bill precisely. It should not be so comfortable that the invitation to fall asleep in it is irresistible; it is hard enough not to do this in any case at certain points in the day. But it should be good enough for one to be able to be as unaware of it as one is of the carpet.

Some therapists have the space for a footstool, a highish one, which contributes to contented survival in later life. The healthiest therapist, whose blood pressure is perfectly normal, will nevertheless develop one of the occupational hazards – swollen ankles at the end of the day – or, to give the unattractive phenomenon its correct name: orthostatic oedema, meaning postural swelling because one's legs hang down. Women are more prone to this than men, as can be observed at any scientific meeting.

Of the two other essentials, one is more obvious than the other. First, heating. This may seem barely worth a mention, but therapists who sit still for hours on end may not appreciate that, for anyone else's taste, the room has become unbearably hot. The second essential is one that is better not to have to learn from experience. One only needs one patient, once in a lifetime, to vomit suddenly, without being able to rush from the room, to realize the advantage in having a metal waste-paper bin. I did learn from experience. I had been treating a young woman in analysis for about three years, when, after a long summer holiday, she suddenly had a psychotic break, including classical 'first-rank' symptoms, that is, she was deluded, and she had hallucinations. I had just settled down in our first session when she said, very upset, that she had broken up with her boyfriend during the holiday, and that people were saying a lot about her, and him, on the television. My blood ran cold. I asked her what sort of things were being said, and how often: 'Oh, terrible things about our relationship, on all the news programmes. And they're *not true*. People in the streets are talking about us, too, and I noticed that all the car numbers on the way here were adding up to the same message.' 'What message?', I asked. 'That he's got someone else. But I'm sure he hasn't, because he talks to me too, and he says not.' I decided to medicate her myself, and try to continue the analysis for a while. She started taking hard drugs as well as the ones I prescribed, and they made her very confused and high and ill. One day, without any warning at all, she shot up on the couch, saying, 'I'm going to be sick!' and violently was. I leapt for the waste bin and shoved it under her face, and we prevented most of the mess there might easily have been.

Other subjects which deserve careful thought, and which may at first appear to be trivia until one has lived with them daily for a few years, include pictures, books, personal bric-à-brac, tissues for the patient, and a rug on the couch.

There is no accounting for tastes, so I can only speak from what my own experience has taught me about surviving with maximum peace of mind. I cannot see the value in arguments which say one should not provide tissues and a rug on the couch for patients' use; there is an austere school of thought, however, which does not provide them. My own feeling is that one is inviting a patient into one's own setting for a possibly painful form of treatment, for which he/she is probably paying a considerable sum of money; I prefer to make this setting as pleasant as may be for both of us. What it boils down to is that *I* feel more at ease if these things are there rather than not. Similarly, I would hate to have a telephone which rang in the consulting room, even if an answering machine deals with the call – which I also regard as near-essential – in another room.

People differ widely on the pictures, books, and personal bric-à-brac question. I only wish to draw attention to the fact that they all need careful thought. I like to have some pictures in the room, and they can certainly evoke valuable transference reactions ('What ghastly taste you've got! I don't know whether I can bear that picture for the next 'x' years.' Or, 'I just love that picture; I can see so much in it, it reminds me of . . .', and so on). The only aspect of pictures which I feel strongly about is that I might have survived my own analysis, at times, with a little less distraction if there had *not* been an evocative picture that hung so I faced it directly from the couch. I think a bare wall allows for freer fantasy in the patient; and I would certainly always choose to have white walls as my personal preference.

The question of clothes is often raised, and these too are part of the daily setting. Indeed, we probably live in more intimate contact with our clothes than with anything else; therefore, it is essential to be comfortable and feel 'right' enough in them that one can forget them. A therapist who is obviously self-conscious, in either an anxious or a narcissistic way, about her clothes, would be quite off-putting to a patient, who might not feel able to broach the subject for a long time.

Readers must allow for the fact that I belong to the generation which never became as adapted to casual clothes as the younger generations have. This no doubt affects my taste and opinions about others, but I have noticed, time and time again, when attending or speaking to audiences of therapists, social workers, and counsellors, that I am not just an old-fashioned creature because I always wear a dress and decent shoes to work in. If I am giving a paper at the end of a day, and people have on the whole come from work, they too, whatever their ages, tend to wear 'good' clothes – dresses, suits, or blouses and skirts; and the men wear suits, or good trousers and jacket, and usually a tie. If I give a paper or go to a lecture on a Saturday, far more people of both sexes turn up in jeans, sweatshirts, and trainers. This suggests to me that there is an unspoken assumption throughout the profession that comfortable, well-adapted clothes are usually meant for work, but not trousers (on women) or jeans or old sweaters, or anything too casual, for either sex. My generation of women tend to wear makeup, though younger women do not; being well-groomed, with clean and tidy hair, does seem to me to be important, and I guess that most people, of both sexes, feel the same.

The management of the practice plunges into technique, so we must remember I am addressing only those features of one's technique which are so much a part of one, that most of the time they probably are not noticeable to oneself, and certainly not to the patient, or not when they have a few sessions behind them. This is not a lengthy study of all aspects of technique, but there are certain things which recur every day of one's working life, and surviving with a relaxed and easy mind depends on getting them right – for oneself. There is no moral right or wrong about most of these things; but there certainly is a 'right' for oneself.

There should be both a lavatory and a waiting area (preferably a room) for patients' use. Ideally, the waiting room should not be full of personal clutter, but a cluttered room is still better than nothing, or just a hall corridor. For a comfortable, successful practice, a lavatory and a good waiting area are essential.

First on the daily list is greeting the patient, who has used some customary way of getting into one's house, and is now in the waiting room. Opinions on one's regular way of getting the patient from there into the consulting room show an astonishingly wide range. At one extreme is a silent glance, barely even a nod, and at the other is a daily handshake, or at least one before every session. I know very few people who are at this latter extreme these days, but Michael Balint and several other European immigrants would have thought anything less to be discourteous. I give a very slight bow and say 'Good morning', or 'Good evening', or whatever it is. My principal objection to the handshake routine – which used to be repeated at the end of every session as well – is that I feel it must interfere with the state of the transference. If I as the patient got off the couch in a state of strong hostility, perhaps in the middle of exploring some angry, negative feelings that had not been hitherto accessible, the last thing I would want to do would be to shake my analyst by the hand. I recall once using this exact phrase to Michael Balint during a seminar. He laughed comfortably and said, 'Well, it *is* the last thing you do . . .'. Clearly his inclination, and therefore personal ease, required this form of behaviour, which I find intrusive to the point of distortion, as well as very controlling.

Having greeted your patient and enabled him, with whatever routine you use, to settle down in the chair or on the couch, how do you continue to 'manage your practice'? How do you give your accounts, and when? Have you made sure that money matters were entirely settled between you before the therapy started? What do you do if the patient fails to pay you? Do you allow the patient to smoke? What do you say if you have to leave the room? What do you say if you are unavoidably late for the session? What do you do if a patient stalks about the room, makes as if to leave, or – in one memorable example of my own - sweeps all the objects off your mantelpiece, including two vases full of water and flowers? (see Chapter 4). How do you handle it if patients meet in the waiting room, or if one stays in the lavatory well into the session-time of the next? How do you tell your patients about dates of holidays, and when? What, if anything, do you say if you make a major change in the setting, for example, if you get a new couch? What do you do if there is a power cut, and it is already dark outside? Would you, under any circumstances whatever, touch a patient?

The subjects touched upon in these questions vary greatly in significance. The point of the whole litany is that sooner or later you will need an immediate answer to some of them, and if they have never crossed your mind, you may find yourself momentarily flummoxed, wishing you had given some thought to whatever the situation is which has suddenly arisen. Of course, survival does not depend on any of them, although perhaps if I include, What do you do if a patient brings a knife and plays idly with it while staring at you? it might.

There are no ready answers to any of these questions, and working on them in seminars with therapists and students I am amazed by the range of views, and the ways in which different people often felt very strongly about their different opinions. From the standpoint of my own survival, I have come to feel more confident through having experienced most of the things brought to mind by the questions.

For example, I fear that I run the risk of forgetting if, and precisely how and when, I have made sure all patients know my holiday dates and have got hold of them firmly. Therefore, about a month before the holiday, I put up a notice in the waiting room giving the exact dates. This way patients often feel they have a few minutes in which to write them down. Certainly all sessions on the day on which I put up the notice tend to produce reactions; but at least I can be ready for that, and my mind is at rest and not having to deal with a faint doubt that I may not have found the opportunity to say it clearly, or at all.

A quantity of emotion of all sorts attaches to money, and the question of payment deserves fuller attention. It is important to discuss the subject in the preliminary interview, before you embark on a treatment, and it is important to get the terms absolutely clear, so that if mistakes occur, you can be sure they are not due to your own muddle, or lack of explanation of your method. Your fee should either be stated, or, if it is a patient with whom you feel the amount needs negotiation, the subject should be covered and settled first thing. Strong reactions to payment by the patient may well form part of future sessional material, but in the beginning you should both be clear on the fee you will be charging, and your method of presenting your bills.

Some patients ask if you want to be paid in cash. This is a trickier question than some therapists seem to realize as hidden in this question is another: 'Are you the sort of person, like me, who avoids paying tax?' It is therefore unwise just to agree to cash. After all, you are going to be this person's therapist, so you are justified in starting the therapeutic work then and there by saying something like, 'What are your own views on that?', or, 'How do you imagine me answering?' Some patients pay in cash without mentioning that they are going to. I prefer cheques myself, and usually say so at some point.

I tell the patient I will put the bill in an envelope on the table in the consulting room on the first day of each month. Then follows the interesting process whereby you begin to learn what sort of a payer the patient is. On the whole our patients are grateful for what we do, and pay us fairly readily, though they may often grumble or discuss it. Reluctant payers have to be tackled therapeutically, and usually show change within a year or so.

I do not think the younger therapist (by which I mean newer, less experienced, you will remember) finds payment questions easy at first. It is, however, useful to try to toughen up and work through your own difficulties over money as soon as possible. Therapy is not a profession in which you will get rich quick – or even slowly. It should bring in a good, adequate income, but it is here, especially at the beginning, that a sense of vocation is also a support. I don't suggest you ever take on a patient for nothing. But you will undoubtedly take on some, intermittently for many years, who are ill and in need, of interest to you, and not well-off. Provided the interest is there, you will not regret taking on one or two patients at a low fee, enabling them to have therapy when they otherwise could not.

However, if a prospective patient has money, do not be afraid to charge a good fee, as high as the market suggests (ask around) and your conscience can stand. It is wise to set a top fee for yourself at all times, which of course will rise as time passes – as should all your others – as this will save you a lot of inner debate in the unlikely event of being faced with a millionaire. However well worked over, greed is as potent in therapists as in the rest of human nature, and if you know you are not going to charge more than 'x', you can put your mind at rest.

I have only had one therapy patient who left owing me money, and that was paid during an attack of conscience some years later. Adequate, unself-conscious dynamic work on late or non-payment should unravel the knots sufficiently to obtain your fees fairly regularly. If someone leaves without paying, I would guess that the whole therapy, and especially the termination work, has been unsatisfactory to both parties.

I do not allow smoking in the consulting room, nor do I make any exceptions. People who wish to smoke are always surprised, sometimes shocked, and very occasionally outraged, regarding this as highly authoritarian; and perhaps it is, but then we can work with that. On the whole smoking is rarer than it was, and crops up most often in the consultation practice, and many interesting reactions have ensued. There is a by now predictable pattern of body language: a patient who has come for a consultation reaches a difficult passage in what needs to be said, usually thirty minutes into the consultation. Sometimes embarking on saying something, sometimes crying, the patient will automatically start patting his pockets, or reach down for her handbag. Sometimes they get as far as extracting a cigarette, even putting it into their mouths, when they suddenly become aware of what they are doing. The conversation then goes like this:

P: 'Oh – you don't mind if I smoke, do you?'
NC: 'Yes.'
P: 'Thanks.' (Often starts to light up, then does a double-take.) 'What did you say?'
NC: 'I said "yes".'
P: 'Yes I may smoke?'
NC: 'No. Yes, I do mind if you smoke.'
P: 'Oh, you do?' (Beginning to show the first signs of being put out.) 'Why?'
NC: 'Because this is a small room, and a lot of people, who have yet to come today, don't like it, and neither do I.'
P: (Now either angry or perhaps pitifully crying, the tone depending on which.) 'But – but – I can't go on if I don't. I always smoke when things get really difficult, I'm feeling dreadfully anxious, don't you understand?'

NC: 'Well, we've got plenty of time, and this is the best place to bring your anxiety.'

Up to this point the conversation is exactly predictable, and has been repeated probably dozens, possibly hundreds, of times. There is, however, a type of patient who will accept what you say gracefully (or compliantly, or masochistically?), and put the cigarettes away, quite agreeable to getting on with the interview without smoking. With these, the conversation stops earlier. With the ones who are really upset and annoyed, it may take a variety of forms from here. I have become convinced by now that there is a coded message about prognosis in these behaviour patterns. I followed up about twenty people – that is, asked for news of the therapy from their therapists from time to time – and whatever one may think about its meaning, it seemed that the patients who took the no-smoking point without rancour consistently did better as a result of treatment than the ones who got upset.

The only person who ever defied it completely was a plain, fractious, unhappy social worker in her fifties, who had three failed treatments behind her already. Her response to my refusal was to become angry and argumentative, though initially she put her cigarettes away. She continued to protest, however, and after about ten minutes said, 'I don't care what you say – I'm *going* to smoke.', and proceeded to do so. This was one of those occasions when I was put on a spot. It had not happened before, so I sat quietly and looked at her, while she smoked furiously, gazing back at me with a mixture of triumph and fear. After a while I said, 'Do you make a habit of getting across people?' She looked taken aback, and then said, 'Well, perhaps I do. So why do you think I do that?', and took out another cigarette. I said, 'It feels as if you're trying to prove that you can beat me on my own ground, but I don't believe you're enjoying it.' 'Oh, I am.' she said at once, unconvincingly, adding, 'I bet I've upset you.' I wasn't exactly upset, but I found myself disliking her, and thinking that she was behaving like a defiant six-year-old. I said, 'You came here looking for a therapy referral, but you must be demonstrating to me something about why your other therapies didn't work. Perhaps you're more interested in spoiling things than in getting better.' She was struck by this, and the interview became more reflective, less contentious, and she did not light a third cigarette. With some misgivings I referred her to a colleague of mine experienced in working with adolescents, who could tolerate acting-out, of which

I warned her there might be plenty. This turned out to be correct, and although the patient stayed for a year – longer than she ever had before - she fought every inch of the way, and acted out over paying, attending punctually, and in other ways.

Although I smoke myself, the reason I give for banning it in the consulting room is the true one, and I long since decided I would never smoke while I was working. I know very well that smoking is not good for people, and I believe it is more appropriate for a doctor not to smoke in public, especially before patients. This has never been a particular hardship, and I am now glad I blocked the possibility for myself of smoking for many hours of every day.

Other points about the management of the practice that should be clarified include names, interruptions, and presents. As to names, there has been a distinct cultural change during the last couple of decades. Apart from the introduction of the unpronounceable 'Ms', which I rarely use, the practice of calling anyone and everyone straightaway by their first names has become widespread.

I do not care to be addressed by my first name on earliest acquaintance. Relatively often people telephone me when they have been referred for assessment, and if I happen to answer the telephone myself, and a cheerful voice says, 'Oh, is that Nina?' I reply, equally cheerfully, 'Yes, who's that?' When the response turns out to be, 'Well, you don't know me, but I've been recommended to ring you, because . . . etc.', my manner changes abruptly. I become cool – I might even say frosty – and even if I do not refer to it at once, the conversation proceeds on rather icy lines. Very often, I will take an early opportunity of asking the caller's age: the use of my first name seems to be in some direct ratio to the speaker's youth. If the answer is 'Nineteen', I will say I do not see young people nowadays (quite true), but that I will refer them on to a colleague of mine who is experienced in working with the young, and then do so. If the caller says they are in their thirties, or even more (at forty or over the habit is much rarer), I say I prefer to be addressed as Dr Coltart by someone who I have not even met yet. The suppressed reaction – 'Stuffy old bag', or 'Pompous git' is frequently almost audible, but that's all right by me. On occasions when we have not previously spoken on the telephone, but have corresponded over the appointment, the same sequence sometimes happens when I first meet the person at the door; there I say my operative bit a little sooner.

My habit is to address people formally when I take them into treatment, and since for about fifteen years I have chosen mostly to treat people well over forty, they do not have difficulty in doing the same to me. Students often call their analysts and training therapists by their first names, or by nicknames, when chatting about them behind their backs, but this is an age-old tradition, and is only a little bit of harmless acting-out. Very rarely, quite late in a long treatment, and with someone younger than myself, I may from time to time call them by their first names. This is quite a complex event, and certainly one has to have thought about it and feel comfortable with it. It usually happens with rather schizoid or borderline people, and is invariably by then welcomed as a particularly personal and private celebration of things between us.

Interruptions to a working session should be kept to a minimum if one has any control over that sort of thing, for example, gas men and electricity-meter readers will usually come early if specifically asked to do so. When an unavoidable interruption occurs, say, a ring at the door when no one else is available to answer, these should be dealt with through the entryphone (a most valuable addition to the therapist's tool kit). At the worst, one will have to get up and go to the front door. If this becomes necessary, I say, 'Excuse me, I shall have to deal with that; I'll be back as soon as I can.' Close the door behind you as you leave the room. Immediately on return, I believe it is correct to invite associations to being left alone in the room. This often produces a wealth of most valuable material: fears of being lost or forgotten; actual memories of such happenings; fantasies of looking in my diary, my cupboards, or desk drawers, if there are any in the room. Some patients, bolder than others, will get up and wander, or stand looking at the books. Such is the power of transference that they will invariably anticipate some sort of ticking-off for behaving like this, and good dynamic work can ensue. So there is nothing to panic about if leaving the room becomes a necessity; such events can always be turned to the advantage of the ongoing therapy.

I do not think one should have a telephone in the consulting room; it is extremely distracting and invasive to a patient – and to the therapist – if it rings and a conversation takes place, however brief. Furthermore, there is no possible excuse for a telephone in this quiet and private place. Answerphones operate everywhere now; and because the telephone usually rings a few times, and then the machine makes other noises, the answerphone itself should be in another room. It can be a great servant and protector to a busy therapist; how anyone could exist without one now is beyond my imagination.

Occasionally patients will bring you presents. Awkward and rejecting though it may seem, there is a strong theoretical rationale for refusing them. They have many layers of subtle meaning, some or all of which can be elicited with careful analysis once the outrage in the patient occasioned by the rejection has been partly worked through. However, like all rules, this one too is made to be broken at times; individual clinical judgement of each and every case must be one's final arbiter. Very occasionally I accept a present which has arisen out of some highly significant piece of work, brought to a successful conclusion, and for which the present may be a tiny symbol. Or the feelings of celebration may be so strong between the therapeutic pair that a present can be accepted with grace.[1] The general rule is not to, the exceptions are rare, and they test one's clinical powers to the utmost.

The only time when I consistently accept a present is at the end of a long treatment. There is unlikely to be a present if the therapy was not a success; if it was, the transference should have diminished considerably by the end, and the therapist is more fully regarded as a separate person with his or her own character. In this guise of one human being relating to another, albeit still in an asymmetrical way, I think it would be churlish to refuse a present which, among other things, expresses some of the patient's genuine gratitude. The acceptance of a present from the hands of a person whom one has accompanied through so many strange, often dark, stages on his or her life's journey can be quite a moving moment. One is by now far removed from that long-distant preliminary interview, and there is a sense of ceremonial closure of one of the most complex, committed relationships of the patient's life. It seems fitting that one should mark such a significant occasion by a unique exchange.

It is probably clear by now that there are few specific rules for handling the many situations that may arise, but that attention to these possibilities means that one can be prepared rather than taken by surprise. Giving an example of my own ways of coping is not intended to imply that these are the only ways, only to provide a few ideas – as in having a couple of candles and some matches somewhere in the consulting room in case of power cuts. Who knows? There may come a day when a sentence or two from this book will swim suddenly into your mind at a critical moment.

4
Paradoxes

The appreciation of the numerous paradoxes in our lives is in itself a survival device. Not only does paradox turn up everywhere in how we live and work, but if we do not see and fully accept it, we deprive ourselves of a whole dimension of enjoyment, and – I think – of skill. Also, we may become confused, feeling inarticulately. 'Oh, I can't do this *and* that', or, '*This* seems to be quite incompatible with *that*; how can I allow for both?' Seeking out, spotting, and tolerating paradoxes is essential to our peace of mind.

I sometimes come across young analysts who have not yet grasped the paradox principle, and who are worried because they feel they are frauds. For them – and at times, for many of us – it seems as if it were somehow sinful to have *needed* one's personal analysis, which is the basic plank in the whole training structure. Here we are, now qualified, setting ourselves up as people who are thought by potential patients to be wise and trustworthy, armed with skills which will assist them to unravel their problems. Yet *we* know we are still anxious, still prone to fright and uncertainty and depression, and that all the difficulties we took to our own analyses, though better and more manageable – some even disappeared – can still beset us. At the end of the training, we are maximally aware of just how unpractised we are, and just how little we know. We haven't even read the whole of Freud *once* yet; and look at all that stuff continually pouring forth from the journals; and we haven't got time to read one-hundredth of it; and it all seems so different actually in the consulting room, and . . .

I would be far more concerned about the professional future of a recently qualified ex-student who *didn't* feel like this. Someone who comes into an analysis without a strong sense of personal need, and who does not experience it as congenial, is not likely to make a good therapist at the other end of it. To emerge from the training brimming with self-confidence, sure that one has the answers both for oneself and for one's patients, is to give a strong impression that one does not even know the questions yet. We approach the paradox at the heart of the matter: psychotherapists are trained from their weaknesses; all other professions build on their strengths.

A 'normal' person is unlikely to be accepted for one of the dynamic therapy trainings. Let us try to define a 'normal' person: someone whose whole defence system is tough and works for him; who clearly has ego strength, does not suffer much, if at all, from anxiety; who feels no interest in introspection, gains little from it, and may well deny he has an unconscious mind; whose emotions are limited, but genuine and likeable; whose life pattern conforms to conventional requirements; and whose temperament is equable and not burdened with emotional swings, impulses, symptoms, or over-dependence on others.

This is a bit of a caricature, but not an extreme one. Would you wish to speak, maybe unhappily and of your most intimate thoughts, to such a person? I wouldn't. I would feel there would be no empathy with my irrational bouts of anxiety, patches of helpless depression, odd symptoms; I would expect to encounter complete bafflement at severe psychological illness. Furthermore, I would be apprehensive that he would 'counsel' me – give me practical suggestions as to how to 'pull myself together', or interrupt me if I sought stammeringly for words to try to express the unthought known. I would be afraid he or she would feel confident they had an Answer (do they even know the Question?).

In many walks of life, when we approach an 'expert' for 'advice', we want answers. If I go to a lawyer, or an architect, or a shoemaker, I don't want to be asked if I have any further thoughts about what I've just said. I want to be told something, have my request treated pragmatically by someone who I expect to know more than I do about the subject. This is where the paradoxes of our profession begin to manifest more clearly. However much we feel anxious, empty of facts, and unable to advise, we *do* know something about how to listen, both to and beyond what is being said. We do know, and we shall soon know more, about how to recognize that what is being unconsciously sought is not always what is being consciously asked; how to remain silent when our words would be superfluous, defensive, or misdirected; and how to acknowledge, both to ourselves and maybe to the other person, that we *don't know the answer*, but that we have faith that our way of being with him is a way that will help him on his path towards knowing himself better, and trusting his own capacities to feel better with that knowledge.

For if we inspect ourselves after our own analyses – perhaps not at once, because the immediate post-analytic phase is often full of sadness and turmoil – we shall realize that though we may still be aware of the capacity for anxiety, depression, and confusion, we have learned different ways of handling these, new ways of staying with 'it', whatever 'it' is, and working through to a better place; that we do, in short, feel 'better' ourselves, and more able for our task. And that we know something about the unique process by which this often quite radically different state was arrived at, though we may not be able to describe it in detail.

Having observed this first great paradox, that it is because we can be anxious, for example, that we can constructively approach someone else's anxiety, we begin to see that in the matters of technique, paradoxes crop up all over the place, and the sooner we learn to exploit this, the better. This is best achieved by confronting the need to create and use a healthy split in our minds; this is the only way we will learn to deploy two paradoxically contrasting states of being, and two sorts of technical achievement, *at one and the same time*. There is nothing acutely paradoxical in doing one thing one day and a different thing in a similar situation on another day. But to be deploying creatively two contrasting attitudes at once is the secret of a skilful technique.

Embedded in our vast literature, these qualities are all somewhere either described directly or, more often, implied. If one tried to make a list of technical skills by reading 200 papers, one would end up in a sorry mess, especially as therapists stress different aspects of technique. It is the vital 'trick of the mind' involved in the splitting – like riding two horses at once, a foot on each – which gives us confidence in our technical flexibility.

I will consider first the most glaring paradox, one which is rarely directly addressed, but is assumed to have been taken in by some sort of osmosis from the atmosphere of a training organization, from our knowledge of other therapists, and from the literature.

With every patient, we embark upon a complex and unique relationship, which may develop and deepen over several years. It is then, in an apparently arbitrary way, quite unlike any other relationship, brought rather starkly to an end. By the time we begin one of these relationships, it is assumed that we are aware that we play our part in it abstinently; 'abstinence' was Freud's word, and there is no reason to modify it today.

The ethics of our profession are strong, clear, and have *raisons d'être*. The only problem is that they are not agreed upon in an internationally accepted formulation. Maybe, leaving it to each one of us to work them out and maintain them, is treating us – and particularly us as students – as responsible, morally aware adults. The ethics of our profession can be summarized, I think, by saying that we should not exploit our patients, especially considering the vulnerability and strength of transference relationships, in any way – emotionally, behaviourally, sexually, or financially.

Strict analytical therapy trainings assume we do not touch our patients, although touching is not so frowned upon in some quarters as in others. Personally, I think touching is always so charged with possible meanings that we simply should not do it. But – and here is our own big professional paradox – it is also assumed that to do effective therapy we allow our own feelings full play, to learn from them in the counter-transference as much as we can about how this patient uses his objects, i.e., us. In our close empathic attention to the patient, we therefore experience the gamut of emotions about and towards him. In order to deploy our best therapeutic selves, we need to be detached observers, coolly appraising every nuance of what happens, *and* at the same time emotionally alive to, and thus involved in, these nuances. A paradox indeed, possible only if we can fruitfully effect the 'trick' of genuinely being two things at once.

Many of the other technical paradoxes are like small-mirror reflections of that first and most important one, referring in more detail to one or other special feature of how we work as therapists. We need to pay detailed attention to everything that is said and every fractional change in the patient's voice, mood, demeanour, behaviour, and material; at the same time, we must scan what is going on as part of a much greater whole, occurring as a tiny moment in a long and complex history. We need to study the state of the transference in particular as it ebbs and flows in the space of one session. But at the same time we must take soundings from the countertransference feelings, which, interwoven with the cool appraisal, tell us not only how we are reacting, but also how we may be experiencing bits of unconscious projection, or projective identifications, from the patient, which, in the welter of things going on, may need to be decoded and handed back to the patient as our primary task.

Then there is the delicate assessment required to decide what we know, and whether to transmit it, as opposed to the (usually stronger) feeling of what we don't know, and why not, and are we in fact meant to be not-knowing as a transference manoeuvre, or is it just us being ignorant? This joins so seamlessly on to the whole business of speaking that I shall consider that next.

Interpreting could be written about at enormous length – and indeed, has been. From our standpoint of examining the enjoyment of paradox, it is necessary to see that we could probably always say more than we do. With a speaking patient – as opposed to a silent one – in one compartment of our minds we need to imagine various things that at any moment we could be interpreting or commenting on; to be rehearsing, scanning possible ways of putting a telling point, selecting a key word, reflecting on a dream interpretation, and so on. At the same time, from the 'other' compartment, we must continue to be attentively with the patient, and finally to decide, probably at some preconscious level, what we are actually going to say, say it, and immediately attend to the response. The subtle pleasures of interpreting, which at one level only is our chief function, are very rewarding, and part of the survival-enjoyment of the therapist.

The last paradox I want to consider is that of the curiously impersonal way we are required to work, with our full self-expression throttled back to a near-minimum. When seen in conjunction with the great power which is ascribed to us in the transference, this is an extraordinary phenomenon.

It is essential for our psychic health that we do not get caught up into semi-delusional ideas that, just because our patients, who are deep in emotional processes, think we are wonderful – or hateful, or cold, or brilliant – we really, secretly, *are* these things. Especially I've noticed, the positive ones. It is necessary for the patient to go through these states of misapprehending us. It was Freud's greatest discovery that this was valuable, not alarming or mad, and that it could be used creatively by the analytic pair. But the paradoxical effect of seeing exactly what the patient means, and where he is, alongside knowing that we are still *us* – ignorant, anxious, striving, waiting, thinking, reflecting – in our own, ordinary ways, can be quite hard to assimilate fully and be relaxed with. Also, we cannot be as spontaneous and emotionally expressive as in any other situation, though analytic spontaneity grows with practice, and is a skill to be aimed for.

Bion's admonition that one should embark on each session 'without memory and without desire' speaks to my theme of splitting the mind in the service of one's technique. It may be objected, for example, 'But I can't *not* have my memory of this patient and his history, and what things are like for him now.' Bion knew that perfectly well. But he also knew that one can hold all that knowledge in suspension as it were, knowing it with one section of one's mind, ready to dip into it at any moment, and, at one and the same time, turning a 'clean surface' of the self towards the patient, poised to receive whatever is conveyed that day, then and there, giving it one's full attention in the here and now. That attention will then be as uncluttered as possible, *informed* by memory, but functionally free of it. It will also be free of 'desire', by which I understand that one must try to leave aside any wishes or hopes or expectations one may otherwise have for this patient, and how he should be in the here and now and in the future.

It is a hard task, and yet one will survive with more integrity and less undesirable influence on the patient if one constantly works towards transcending all wishes, hopes, expectations, plans, advice, and what we think best for this person. Only thus can we survive, knowing in our bones that the patient will be able to leave us ultimately as fully himself as we have been able to allow to him, unpushed, undistorted by anything that we might happen to think good or bad for him, responsible for himself, his choices and his decisions, his own thinking – his Self, in fact.

The hardest thing about this task – and yet perhaps the most vital – is to pare away any ambition we may have that he get 'better'. *Our* ideas about what 'better' means for the patient are necessarily conditioned by our own world-views, and these may not be what the patient needs at all. He may even for his own reasons prefer to remain ill, or anxious, or symptomatic. There may be strong secondary gains in it for him.

The suicide of a patient, which many therapists may have to endure at least once, is a very hard experience, which brings to the fore with singular clarity what a tightrope we are on as we do our balancing act: we need to be able to trust that we did everything we were capable of, yet to accept that that was not enough; at the same time we have to respect the patient's final responsibility for himself. It may be that the single-minded strength of his determination to kill himself out-manoeuvres all our therapeutic skills, and in the last resort we may have to accept the inner logic of his decision. Our hopes, our good will, and our professional pride may be badly damaged, but it is important not to exaggerate any guilt that may be a cloak for our wounded narcissism.

I have seen very little literature about suicide in patients who are undergoing therapy or analysis, which I suspect is to do with a complex of reasons that include a somewhat alarming and taboo quality surrounding the subject. However that may be, threats of suicide, either hysterical or severely depressive, are not uncommon in our work, and many older therapists have a memory of one successful suicide in their practices.

As suicide is probably the worst hazard of the kind of work we undertake, and since it is profoundly distressing for a therapist, I think it is something that should be looked at in some detail. It has to be survived, the practice with many other patients has to go on, with the therapist's self-confidence and individual attention to those patients as intact and resourceful as possible.

A patient who kills him/herself is the ultimate paradox in our working lives. The aim of our therapies could be defined as increasing the wellbeing and the (relative) happiness of the people who come to us for help. Healthy and enjoyable survival of the therapist implies that the self-esteem accruing from the months and years of patient endeavour to alleviate psychic suffering should be solid and supportive to ourselves. From whatever angle one studies it, one cannot escape the stark knowledge that suicide stands for failure.

There is even something 'not quite nice' in considering the suffering of the therapist at all in this context. When a person dies in unhappy circumstances, there is anger and a natural tendency to look around for someone to blame; and if the dead person died in circumstances which involve medical or professional care, the most obvious person to blame is the physician, surgeon – or therapist. Patients who have been severely depressed, with maybe psychotic intensity for a long period, may well have alienated relatives who are not informed or enthusiastic about analytical therapy in the first place; if this person kills him/herself during the therapy, it is remarkable how the alienation is forgotten as the fury, fuelled by guilt, is directed by nearest and dearest at the unhappy therapist, who may well have struggled against overwhelming odds.

This is most especially the case with the young hysteric. There are a number of young patients, predominantly women, who are part of the in-and-out population of psychiatric units, and who make a professional career of slashing and overdosing. Normally they do not come into regular dynamic therapy, but many of us will have treated them, or at least one, when we ourselves were young. These patients are the type who 'die in the attempt'. They do not really intend to 'die'; their problem is that they do not know how to live. Their muddled young minds have no grip on managing life, or how to see a way through the mess they are in. They usually come from 'socially deprived' backgrounds, and they are said to be uttering 'cries for help' as they cut their arms or swallow a dozen paracetamol tablets. I do not mean to be dismissive – they *are* in a mess, and they *are* sending out cries for help. The trouble from our end is that we are not infinitely resourceful, though it may have been conveyed to the public that we are. There is a pretty strict limit to the help which can be offered, and, moreover, there may be an even narrower limit to how much of our sort of help such people can assimilate.

Since our resources are limited in more than one way, we have to exercise judgement about the patients we undertake to treat by means of analytical therapy. It is here that diagnosis and assessment comes into its own, and the need for selectivity underpins the emphasis I have put on psychological-mindedness (see Chapter 6).

It does not become us to proclaim that, as everyone is equal and has equal rights, everyone should have the chance, if required or requested, of experiencing psychotherapy. This viewpoint may well be Politically Correct, and reflect some virtuous glow on its proclaimer, but such a one is responding to cultural conditioning, and not to the dictates of wisdom, or even to common sense. Quite apart from whatever views one may hold on the question of people's rights, we are not being fundamentally honest, and we are certainly not looking after our own healthy survival, if we make out that we can and should offer treatment to anyone at all, regardless of their type of disorder, capacity for responsible introspection, and informed wish to work at the kind of therapy we have been trained to offer. To behave as if – even worse, to believe that – we can treat anyone and anything with a hope of providing real help is to be caught into omnipotence, and the idealization both of psychoanalysis and of ourselves.

In the early 1970s, a forty-seven-year-old woman was referred to me by her GP, who worked in a provincial town, but told me in his letter that the patient was prepared to travel to London twice a week if I could offer her therapy. She was very attached to this GP, and often visited him with irregular somatic symptoms and constant complaints of depression. Just as constantly, he had suggested she would benefit from some psychological help, and finally got her to agree. The woman presented a mixed picture from the beginning. Ostensibly, she refused to contemplate the possibility that psychotherapy would be of any use; at the same time, she presented a marked and subtle psychological-mindedness.

She had been the sort of thoroughly intelligent, rather bookish, working-class girl who had to leave school when she was sixteen, but would have repaid a hundredfold the chance of further education, which only became possible in this country some years after she had embarked on adult working life. She was plain, tough, and humorous, and I imagined she had been quite frightening to boys of her own age at a time when her few friends were getting married and starting families. She had a salty, ironic way of talking, which, together with her psychological acumen, made her an attractive proposition for twice-weekly psychotherapy. From the beginning I took to her and found her easy to like, which was just as well as she soon revealed that she needed to enact a drama with me in which unrelenting hatred of her mother informed one layer of the transference for months on end.

In herself and in her transference she presented a striking example of paradox. She was extremely scornful about men, whom she regarded as weak and useless; at the same time, she had been desperate to get married, at a time when it was not fashionable among the young to go to a dating agency or marriage bureau, as such organizations were then more commonly called. It will be remembered that she adored the referring GP, a tall, handsome, masculine man. She had met her husband, who I will call Tom, through a bureau. They fell deeply in love, and had been married for about eighteen years. Neither wanted any children. They still loved each other as much as ever.

Continuing the theme of paradox, she stated firmly – and for three years did not waver from this stated view – that her mother was 'a monster; quite simply, a monster. Diabolical, she was.' Yet she soon became emotionally attached to me in a passionate, devoted way, which, though she concealed it as much as she could, showed a capacity for loving women as well as men which had not sprung into being only with her therapy. She poured scorn on almost everything I said from the very beginning, yet she was always punctual for her appointments, never complained about the long, complicated journey she had to undertake to reach me, and, in her blackly humorous way, indicated she understood and absorbed interpretation. A typical exchange between us went like this:

P: 'So, what are we going to talk about today? *I've* got nothing to say to you. It's up to you.'
NC: 'I expect you've been thinking about what we said last time, all the same.'
P: (Indifferently) 'I can't even remember what we said last time. I've got more to think about than you, you know.'

NC: 'Such as?'

P: 'Well, my wretched sister phoned. I can't think why. She knows I've got nothing to say to her . . .'

NC: 'Either?'

P: 'What? What do you mean, *either*? How can I understand you, if you just utter monosyllables?'

NC: 'You haven't anything to say to me, and you haven't anything to say to your sister – either.'

P: 'No, well, I haven't. And trust you to bring yourself in again. That's just *like* my sister, actually; she simply does not seem to accept that I don't like her, I don't want to talk to her, and I'd die happy if I never saw her again. (Pause) I suppose in a minute you're going to remind me that's what I said about my mother last time.'

NC: 'What, exactly?' (The mother had died ten years previously.)

P: 'That I was quite happy never to see her again when she died because I'd felt like that before. Why am I telling you? I pay you to remember what I said last time. (Pause) I did think about you saying you didn't believe me. I don't know how to *make* you believe me, but I'm going to. Can't you understand that I really hated my mother? I did. I was just so relieved when she died. *She* used to say things a bit like you, contradicting me. Oh, she always knew best. Telling me I was lying.'

NC: 'Well, you do. You told me so yourself.'

P: (A bit flustered) 'I know. But that was about *other* sorts of things, to the people at work, nosy parkers. I don't want them knowing all my business; not lying to my *mother*. She must have known I hated her, and didn't want her around.'

NC: 'Yes, but you had other feelings as well, and you knew it; like you do here.'

P: 'I *don't*. Oh, you're so conceited . . .'

This dialogue, which I've actually transcribed from the early days of keeping full notes on the patient, I hope demonstrates both her paradoxical way of being, and the enjoyment we both had in the therapeutic dialogue. I don't intend to convey that the patient was being consciously ironic, or had her tongue in her cheek; she meant exactly what she said, and she said it all in a charged, emotional way, and she glared at me a lot of the time. But there was a mixture of naïvety and psychological sophistication about her – again paradoxical – which was revealing of her disallowed other layers of self.

It was essential to stay closely with the transference work, and not to make it half-humorous, not to appear to conspire jokily with her denials *or* with the hidden and forbidden emotions. The central paradox, I thought, was that this woman was ill, depressed, as a result of splitting off and denying not her negative feelings, rage and hate, as is so often the case with people we see, but her positive feelings – her real capacity for love and tenderness. Her mother, and maybe her weak, drunken father, were monstrous in some unconscious way, because somehow the huge creative energies locked away in this woman's loving feelings had all become blocked and taboo and somewhat shameful. Her only outlet was animals, as well as her husband. He and she ran a smallholding, on which they had chickens, ducks, geese, a few goats, sheep, and pigs, and a cow. She wouldn't have a dog or a cat, 'because I don't want to be tied to the wretched things'. This was ridiculous, as she didn't do anything except go to work. I took it that she meant she didn't want to get so attached to them that she would suffer if they died.

Death was a preoccupation of hers; her humour was macabre and at times violent. She dwelt on both her parents' dying, and their last illnesses. She said, more than once, 'If anything happened to Tom, I'd kill myself.' But she did not threaten suicide at any point. She was a *grande hystérique*, with the dramatic talent that is sometimes associated with this type, but she did not make empty threats. However, I had yet to discover this.

She arrived one day for her session looking grim and haughty. As she sat down opposite me – she had poured scorn on the early offer of the couch – she drew from her handbag a long, sharp-looking, steel knife. For once she did not open the session with some rude provocative remark, but sat staring loftily past me out of the window, revolving the knife slowly in her hands. I watched her, and rapidly examined the possibilities in my mind. I did not think for a moment she had any serious intention of stabbing me, but that she was a creature of some impulse had already been established in the therapy. There had been several minor bits of acting out: she had once torn up a lot of family photographs after showing them to me and scattered them over the floor round her. I said she seemed to be disposing of some family memories into me, her waste bin. I had asked her politely to pick them up before she left, and she had done so. On another occasion, she had thrown a book she had been ambivalent about out of the train window. So I thought, all in all, a minor flesh wound was on the cards.

I wondered whether it would be appropriate to let her know that I appreciated she was in a powerful position; to interpret aggressive or sexual symbolism in the knife itself; to pick up some threads of discussion as if I hadn't noticed; or to stay silent. These were only four possibilities – there were certainly more. They are an example of the sort of decision-making process which is at work in therapists all the time as we reflect on whether to speak, and if so, what to say, and why.

In the end, since it was clearly I who had to speak first, I said, 'I guess you mean to frighten me today.' 'Well, I certainly hope so', she said promptly. She had obviously been longing for this conversation to begin. We discussed at some length how satisfying it would be, branching out into the sense of mute and furious helplessness she had often suffered with her mother. Eventually, after a longish silence, I said, 'I think I'd feel more comfortable if you gave the knife to me for the rest of the session.' 'What, and hand over the power to you?' she said. 'Well, yes, I suppose so. It depends how far you trust me not to use that sort of power', I said. She considered this in silence. Then, somewhat to my surprise, she handed the knife to me, blade first. Rather gingerly I grasped the blade and took it. The session continued.

Some weeks later she was very angry for some reason, which I thought was to do with having enjoyed her previous session and having felt good over the weekend. I said as much. She was furious. The following conversation ensued:

P: 'Oh, you think you're so wonderful. I had a nice weekend because Tom and I did some things we like doing, nothing to do with you. You don't make one *quarter* the difference to me that you seem to think. Tom and I are perfectly capable of enjoying ourselves, always have been.'

NC: (After a short pause) 'I do wonder why you come sometimes.'

P: (Almost hissing with rage) 'Because I'm *depressed.* You know that. I have been for years. Just because I don't go round with a long face, weeping and carrying on all the time . . . I suppose that's what you'd like me to do. Well, I'm not *going* to, just to please you. My mother could make me cry, and I swore when she died no one else ever could. Why, I'd like to make you cry. I – I – I'd - I'd like to *hurt* you.'

NC: 'What, in sort of revenge?'

P: 'Yes. No. I don't know. No, to make you cry. I'll – I'll sweep all those silly things off your mantelpiece. See if you like that.'

NC: (Unwisely, perhaps) 'Well, I wouldn't like it. But I don't think it's the sort of thing that would make me cry – or you, for that matter.'

P: (Now obviously intrigued by her idea) 'I will. I'd really *like* to do that. I bet people don't do things like that. You always think you can control everybody's behaviour, we're all going to be *good* when we come here, and please *you*.'

NC: (Going off rather pointlessly on a different tack) 'You do have a mixed relationship with the other people who come here, don't you, in your mind?'

P: (Perfectly accurately) 'Don't try to change the subject. You think you can just distract me, don't you? We'll see . . .'

Suddenly her impulse overtook our conversation, and, leaping to her feet, she made a broad powerful sweep with her right arm, and swept every single object off my mantelpiece straight at me. (For the sake of those who enjoy detail in their stories, there were two little silver boxes, a filigree basket, two small, fluted silver vases with water with freesias in them, eleven Vermeer postcards, a glass dish with a few paper clips in it, and a carriage clock – see 'Apparent Trivia', Chapter 3! There was also a small but elaborately carved piece of ivory netsuke, a Japanese lady which was elegantly made in four pieces.)

I sat and dripped amidst the wreckage. The carriage clock was in my lap, and the head of the Japanese lady, I was secretly delighted to see, had rolled towards the patient. In the excitement of the moment, and propelled towards me by the thrust of her arm, she stood over me six inches from my knees and spat out triumphantly, 'There! You minded, *didn't you*? You've blushed.' I do blush easily, and I'm sure she was right. I said, in an aggravatingly mild voice, 'Yes, of course I minded. I said I would.'

She turned to go back to her chair. As she did so, she saw the head of the Japanese lady. She was instantly horrified. I felt quite sorry for her; it ruined her moment of triumphant power. She and Tom genuinely loved and collected small antiques, and, ironically, her enjoyable weekend had been spent adding to their treasures. 'Oh', she cried, in real sorrow. 'Oh, I've broken your lady. I'm dreadfully sorry. I really didn't mean – oh, how awful.' Tenderly, she picked up the head. I took pity on her. 'It's all right', I said. 'She's made in four separate bits. Help me pick up the things, and I'll show you.' Willingly, she collected up the various objects, and I showed her how the little statue was put together. I fetched a cloth and mopped up the water, and refilled the vases. The session continued.

She had already made strides in her therapy, fiercely kept from me, but it is also true to say that the Mantelpiece Day, as it came to be known, was a crossroads for her. From then on she did not put so much energy into concealing from me the fact that she was deriving benefit from attention of a certain sort, and from insight, and many things about her changed markedly for the better. I don't mean she ceased to be provocative and scornful, but she allowed her humour to show through; she let me know she knew, and knew that I knew she was happier, and that she often said one thing emotionally, and more consciously meant its opposite. The therapy, in which there was certainly a lot to be done, continued fruitfully for three years.

Then Tom, hitherto a strong and healthy man, developed a suspicious mole on his wrist. He had it biopsied, and the diagnosis came back: it was a melanoma of a highly malignant kind. Four months after he had had an extensive excision, he became quite rapidly ill. He was admitted to hospital; he had multiple metastases. There was no treatment save palliative care. He and my patient were determined he should be at home, and his doctors agreed. There he died after five awful weeks, when my patient nursed him tenderly and devotedly throughout, with the help of the excellent local district nurses. My summer holiday unfortunately coincided with most of these weeks, but as I was not going abroad, and as by now I could in no way have disengaged from this patient at such a time, I gave her my address and telephone number. She rang me nearly every night, just for a few minutes, and she wrote to me every day, both before and after Tom's death. Most days I wrote back a few lines.

When I returned to work, my patient came to her sessions as before. Although now in a state of deep mourning, for about four months there was a level of hypomania which made her state of mind, as was so characteristic of her, curiously mixed. She was profoundly bereaved, lonely, and genuinely in mourning; at the same time, she could be extremely funny, sharper and more ironic than she had ever been, and her histrionic gifts enabled her to appreciate her role as the victim of tragedy, and local widow in her country town. There is something bizarrely ironic in saying that her imitations of people who didn't really know how to address her situation made us laugh until we cried (she had wanted to make me cry, you will recall; we realized this was a better way of doing it).

It was a very odd experience for me as I too felt a number of things at one and the same time. I clearly saw the hypomania, which, nevertheless, sustained her. It was my professional job to interpret its workings, she expected me to, and I did – yet I did not want to dismantle too fast the positive power of a tricky psychological mechanism to hold her through her first stages of mourning. I sometimes dreaded the disappearance of the hypomanic assistance, though I knew it to be specious and that it would not last. This I did not say to the patient; perhaps I should have done. The mourning gradually became distanced, and the hypomania became more powerful.

After about three months, she began to make plans. She applied to join the Open University to read humanities. I could not but think that if this could be got under way it would be a strong ally in the survival process for her. She even considered going to South Africa over the following Easter to investigate some geological sites which furnished the stone which was used in making the handles of small paper-knives (knives!) which she had seriously collected for years. I was very suspicious of all this. I could never forget the emphasis with which she had said, long ago, 'If anything happened to Tom, I'd kill myself.' We discussed this often, and at such depth as we could reach, but she was continuously protected by the magic mantle of the hypomania. Nevertheless, I returned to it as often as I could, from whatever angle of intricacy presented itself.

She confided in me shortly before the Christmas break that she had some morphine sulphate tablets which she had been permitted to administer to Tom in the last painful and wretched stages of his illness, and which should have been collected thereafter by 'the authorities' who had let her have them. Short of telling her GP, which I did, I did not see what else I could do, apart from talk about her transference, and real, intentions in giving me this information. I could not arrange for her admission to hospital; she was not 'ill enough' or 'mad enough' for that. Only I could see that buying new clothes and planning a big trip was 'mad' at that point in time in the context of what I knew about her.

She kept in touch through the Christmas holiday, and it was not until about the end of January that our pseudo-ally, the pervasive hypomanic state, deserted her. Then all that I had dreaded descended like the Furies. Whatever the harrowing of Hell was in mythology, the phrase sounded to me descriptive of how life became for her. She looked back upon the preceding five months in disbelief. She came to her now three sessions a week to sit in deep silence which was filled with suffering. Her third session was on a Friday, and each Friday afternoon I sent her a postcard, for her to receive on the Saturday. Her early months of hostility long forgotten, she now said quite openly that only being in touch with me would keep her going through to some more sunlit upland when this agony should, we hoped, be behind her. So we continued for another month.

Then in early March, her GP, my old friend, rang me one day to say that she was dead. She had been found by the curate (she had taken up religion in her manic state), who, curious and persistent when he could get no answer on Monday morning, had got the police, who had managed to effect an entry. She had cut the telephone cord – the cord to me, I suppose, to life and hope – and had wired all the door handles to heavy objects. There was a long letter to me which she had written as she lay tidily in bed dying, the handwriting drifting away towards the end: '...I would...have liked...to...hold your hand...' On the doormat lay my Friday postcard, delivered on that Monday morning. As she had said in her long note, she realized it would be, but its non-arrival on the Saturday had been all (all?) that was needed to tip her over her edge. The letter was delivered to me only after the inquest, when a sympathetic coroner and her good lawyer had made my task – which could have been hard – a light one.

The paradoxes that this patient carried in her personality left their mark on me in a particular way at this point; and yet it is one that in this extreme situation – which I hope none of you has to endure, and yet which comes to many therapists at least once – has its own logic. I knew this woman would be a severe suicidal risk, under a certain set of formerly unanticipated circumstances. I strove in the short term and the long to make it less likely, and to shore up her defences, as well as to broaden her insight, and strengthen her ego and her hope. While I was not surprised when she finally did kill herself, I felt profoundly shocked. It was as if the event was a complete bolt from the blue. It was quite an odd phenomenon; I was made newly aware of the kind of splits, conscious and unconscious, engineered and hidden, that we have to live with in our attitudes to our work. All over again I reflected on Bion's saying that we work, ideally, without memory and without desire. I suppose it is the same as saying that we have to be prepared for anything, and yet have faith that the extraordinary process is worth involving ourselves in.

5
The Pleasures of Assessment

For me, and I am sure for many of my colleagues in the field of psychotherapy, one of the main planks in the survival structure has always been the continual enjoyment to be derived from the work itself. Curiosity is a requisite in the character of a therapist, and this feature is both fed and stimulated in a particularly gratifying way by the regular practice of consultation. A fuller and more descriptive title is diagnosis and assessment and decision-making, with special attention to referral for psychoanalysis or psychotherapy – or *not* because on occasion the decision which is reached concerns the *un*suitability of the person under review for any form of therapy consisting solely of verbal interchange. Sometimes such people need something else, and then the assessor's task is not only to decide with the patient what that something else is, but also, as for referrals for 'talk-therapy', to set it up, or at least to get the patient on his or her way.

Over the long period in which I have done regular assessments, which during the last couple of decades were averaging three or four a week, about five percent of people have fallen into the 'unsuitable' category. The decisions I have reached with them have ranged through referring them to a behaviourist, to discussing 'medication only' with the GP, to working through with them the possibility of abandoning the notion of any sort of treatment, and carrying on from there without help.

Surprisingly often, this last variation is the one most strongly desired by the patient, though it may not have cropped up – consciously at least, or in so many words – during the session. And yet it can secretly be a consummation devoutly to be wished by the patient. There may be an initial flurry of disappointment, real or enacted, or a sense of 'failure' in the patient which connects with the (projected) feelings in the assessor. It is as if the patient has some dim but definite fantasy of our world, in which ideally everyone sooner or later should have therapy. Of course, substance for this fantasy is provided by certain sorts of media presentations, books, and, I regret to say, the opinions of some of our colleagues.

If one is not prescribing anything at all, an essential piece of work is to establish a conviction of the rightness of this in and for the patient. It requires considerable skill to reinforce the often-hidden wish in the patient to be 'let off', and to strengthen his resolve and his ability to take full responsibility for himself. This emphasizes a need for authentic conviction in the assessor that for this person to commit himself to the expensive, dependent process of therapy would be disadvantageous, would be a brake rather than an accelerator on his progress through his life. We have to be so sure that, although it may be a demanding challenge, he both can and should rise to it, and that we can convey this to him in a way which is creative and will be of positive help to him after he has left us. If by any chance – though I find this is rare in people who have selected themselves far enough to have got to me in the first place – the main reason for our decision is that the patient is so totally unpsychologically-minded (see Chapter 6) that the whole process would be simply baffling for both parties, then we have to convey this to the patient, simultaneously reinforcing his self-reliance. It is no better and no worse to be psychologically-minded than not. It is important not to give the patient who we are dissuading from therapy the impression that we think he is 'one down' in comparison with us superior, sensitive creatures.

I find that in cases with a no-treatment outcome, some particular and necessary piece of work may take place during this one session. Sometimes this takes the form of working on a dream which the patient had the preceding night. Often these dreams are volunteered spontaneously in the session; if they are not, it is worth asking if there has been one. For example, a man who did not need treatment, but was sure I would think he did, dreamed that he entered the grounds of a stately home somewhere in Europe, and there was a fête (his fate?) going on. Lots of rather grand, intimidating women tried to make him buy things from their stalls, and were very persuasive and insistent. Though feeling confused and somewhat alarmed, he consistently rejected them, and at last found to his relief that he was walking up a mountain path, alone, and had left the scene of the fête far behind and below him. It was a simple piece of work on this clear dream which convinced him of the strength and validity of his own wish not to embark upon any therapy.

People sometimes are surprisingly dissociated from their dreams, even those who are actually in analytic therapy. It is as if this story, which they have created, does not quite belong to them.

There is a particular comment I quite often have to make, which, considering its brevity and simplicity, is exraordinarily powerful. A patient who has recounted a significant dream may say, after we have discussed and interpreted it, something like, 'But that man was simply talking about what he was being offered at the sale *in the dream*. What has it really to do with anything *we're* talking about?' At which point I say, 'But it was *your dream*.' That's all. It seems to be all that is needed for the true meaning of the dream to click.

Though we may not often encounter them professionally, there are people to whom the very existence, let alone the multiple influences, of the unconscious are simply not comprehensible on any terms. It does not now seem so odd to me as it used to when I was a zealous young student that these people are nevertheless making a pretty good go of their lives! We are so conditioned in the field of analytical therapy to the 'given' that the unconscious not only exists but is extremely powerful, that we may in our enthusiasm consider such people to be far more limited, lumpen, and dull than the reflective, neurotic souls to whom we are accustomed – including, of course, ourselves.

Large numbers of people, who are what may be meant by 'normal', live lives that are contented and reasonably happy most of the time. What else are we trying to achieve with our patients? Some of my best friends are normal. One is a cheerful, equable, and much-loved GP. When she would describe patients who were fractious, or difficult, or seemed to have nothing medical wrong with them, I would comment in sophisticated analytic terms: 'But he's envious of his wife and attacking her by doing so-and-so, *and* projecting his anger and anxiety into her', I would say, rather pompously. This GP would look at me quizzically for a moment, 'Well, of course he is', she would say. 'But the fact remains, *he* won't see that, and *he's* in my surgery every week saying he must have a certificate . . .' I would sigh as I realized that yet again I must inspect my narcissism and the possibility that I was idealizing, making special my new-found knowledge.

The sources of referrals in my consultation practice are many and varied. An important one arises from self-selection. Almost the highest percentage are self-referred, or – which amounts almost to the same thing – have my name suggested to them by ex-patients or ex-consultees. Out of interest I have always tried to track down the source of referral, but nowadays it is as likely as not that the final link in the chain is a name unknown to me.

I am reminded here of a very frequent phenomenon that is also very odd and noticeable. Quite often during a consultation a patient will say 'Oh, I had some therapy a few years ago.' When I ask for how long, it may have been as much as three or four years, or it may only have been a few weeks or a few sessions. Then I ask, 'Who with?' (or, if I am feeling more pedantic, 'With whom?'). I ask not simply out of curiosity, though that may well come into it, but because the answer usually gives me some notion of what sort of therapy this patient may have had, for example, the theoretical background, the likelihood of transference work, the possibility of physical components, whether there may have been any political or religious bias to it and so on. With astonishing frequency, the reply is, 'Oh, it was – er – I can't seem to think of his/her name – I'll think of it in a minute . . .' But they don't. It is so amazingly widespread – between eighty and ninety percent of interviewees – that it must mean something. Severe ambivalence suggests itself; but whether to therapy, or to that person, or about the patient's own wish for treatment, I do not know.

Self-referrals also come from people who have heard me speak somewhere, and a useful feature here is that the patient already has some information about me, which facilitates both the opening phase of the consultation, and some valuable, and often surprising, work on any fantasy they may have built on that information. Of course, fantasy about what I am going to be like also occurs in people who have never seen me, and I do always try to include some examination of this during the interview. It is rarely voluntered spontaneously, and it almost always reveals some valuable psychological data. Numerous examples spring to mind: 'I thought you'd be very little and dark and waspish'; 'Oh, I didn't think you were nearly as old/young/warm/cold as you seem to be'; 'Well, I thought you'd have a foreign accent'; 'Oh – I don't know . . .', but when pressed, for there always is a fantasy with transference features to it, 'Well, you're much bigger/fatter/thinner/more talkative/silent than I thought you'd be.' Perhaps the most unnerving, but fortunately single, example was 'I thought you'd be exactly like my mother – and you *are*.' It is worth doing some quite careful interpretative work, opening up the use of the transference, on such information.

Apart from these self-referred, or rather, self-selected patients, there are referrals from colleagues (analysts and psychotherapists), psychiatrists, GPs, and people working in various institutions, such as mental hospitals, charities, and so on. Poor sources of referral are acquaintances who know little about our field, and doctors who are antagonistic to therapy but are searching for a last resort. There is much to be said about ill-judged referrals, but perhaps it is enough to say that these are usually the patients who are not psychologically-minded, and with whom the whole session is uphill, slogging, and frustrating, who rarely require the sort of treatment which we have to offer, and who are openly relieved when I do not offer it. The straight clinical interest is of course greater with a person who has a complex psychological problem, and whose tale unfolds with a sufficient number of clues to help one to begin to unravel it there and then.

Sometimes I sit back after an intensive two hours, before I begin to write my notes, and think what a stroke of good fortune consultation practice is to me: the constant, absorbing, always-changing, never-repeated series of windows on the world that is offered is a special blessing in a profession which, however satisfying in all its other aspects, does undoubtedly have a restricting effect on one's life. However deeply we are engaged with the lives of the patients who make up our regular practice, they can only be a limited number, and they can only go on living out their story, with which we soon become intimately acquainted. As well, many of them work in fields which are the same as, or closely allied to, our own. Through doing a lot of assessment work, the astonishing and varied procession of strangers passing our way but once offers a different, colourful dimension to the everyday life of a therapist with a full-time practice.

It is with a unique and intensely enjoyable sense of anticipation that I settle back in my chair opposite a person about whom I know precisely nothing, and realize that by the end of the interview I will be the privileged possessor of an entirely new story. It is as good as starting a new novel, and it is far more rare to be disappointed. In fact, it is true to say that it is impossible to be disappointed; even a patient who is boring, or inarticulate, or pompous, or heavily defended, or hostile is, for that two hours, of unparalleled interest. It might be a different matter to have this person in regular therapy, but the very characteristics which could make regular contact difficult or unattractive, are for the space of the consultation time uniquely engaging and fascinating.

I allow plenty of time for an assessment, and I aim to finish my part in what is needed in the one appointment. I evolved a way of doing assessments over the years which could best be described as encountering someone with something problematical going on in their lives, which they or somebody else (usually the latter) recognize as coming roughly into the area of 'psychotherapy', and which needs help with a solution, or help in moving towards a solution.

Referrers have ranged from the over-enthusiastic, and thus counter-productive, to the prejudiced-against, who used me as a sort of last-ditch when everything else had failed or been rejected. The attitudes of referrers strongly affect the 'set' with which the person comes, and in this I include their hopes, fears, fantasies, and overall positive or negative feelings. I know for certain that much thought is devoted by the patient to an appointment which has been made but for which there may be a few weeks to wait. If patients then forget to come, I infer the presence of strong ambivalence; they may have been encouraged to seek help by some well-meaning friend, relative, or professional whose enthusiasm for the idea overwhelms them, and flattens protest, or makes them feel helpless or frightened. There are all sorts of possibilities, but that forgetting is significant cannot be doubted. After about an hour, which is the most that is likely to be due to traffic jams, train delays, and so on, I telephone their home number, which it is important to have obtained when they first rang or wrote to ask for an appointment. There may be no answer, or I may be told 'Oh, no, he's at work. He'll be in about eight pm', or, 'They went on holiday yesterday.' This postpones the detective work for a time. But surprisingly often the missing person answers. This is where my part in constructing the pattern gets under way. The conversation frequently goes something like this:

NC: 'Is that Mr/Mrs X?'
P: 'Yes, speaking.'
NC: 'This is Dr Coltart here.'
P: 'Oh *hallo*! How are you?'
NC: 'I'm fine, thank you. How are *you*?'
P: 'Oh, keeping well – yes, thanks.'
NC: 'I was wondering where you were.'
P: 'Er – were you? Um – well – oh, heavens! What's the date? Oh, my God, it's not – the eighteenth. I'm meant to be seeing you . . .'
NC: 'Yes.' (This response is cool, but at the same time rooted in interest, though not overdone.)

From here on, there are a number of variations, the most frequent of which is:

P: 'Gosh, how awful. I *am* so sorry. I was so sure it was next
        week/Thursday/September . . .'
NC: (After a pause) 'Do you think maybe it says anything about
        your not wanting to come?'

The responses to this can be informative, and may again branch
out in different directions, from an immediate grasp of the point to
a flurry of anxious denials. I then ask if they would like to make
another appointment, though adding that, regrettably, there will
be another few weeks' wait, and I shall be obliged to charge for
this missed appointment.

Patients' reactions to the second point sort out the sheep from
the goats. Some people are immediately annoyed, hurt, outraged,
and lose no time in expressing these feelings. These are the truly
ambivalent ones, though their negative feelings about coming may
be rooted in fear. Others say at once that they quite understand, of
course they have wasted my time, and they would like another
appointment, but will put a cheque in the post for this one. Whatever one's views on meekness, passivity, over-adaptation, anxiety
to please, one has to admit that these people are socially more
agreeable, make it easier for me to overcome my own feelings of
annoyance (for they *have* wasted my time; there is little else I can
do with that two hours). They are probably more depressed, but
less ill, than the outraged ones, and in the long run more likely to
take to analytical psychotherapy and use it. (They compare inter-
estingly in this way with a certain sort of smoker, referred to in
Chapter 3.) This seems a large edifice to build on such a small
foundation, but there have been enough of such happenings, with
sufficient information later, to warrant this clinical view. And the
consultation as an event-in-itself hasn't even started yet.

Careful follow-up indicates that the people who take most readily to the analytical-therapy way of working and – what is perhaps
more important – need it, and are suitable for it (see Chapter 6) are
those who are referred by ex-patients. The ratio is almost 100
percent exact. This is in quite strong contrast to those referred by
psychoanalysts, other psychotherapists, NHS consultants, and
self-referrals. On the whole, GPs make good referrers. I regularly
place a small number of GP referrals in full analysis each year, and
there are certain GPs whose patients I look forward to seeing in a
particular way, knowing that they will be ill, psychologically-
minded, and ready and willing for treatment. I am acquainted with
a small number of GPs who write full and rich referral letters, spot

exactly the right patients at the right time (often having nursed them along for several years until the exact moment of readiness), and who may have had some therapy themselves, may even have seen me in the past for their own personal assessments and referrals. There are also some others who do good 'old-fashioned' medicine with their patients, knowing their families and life stories, talking and listening to them, not too bothered about the level of their serum rhubarb, but very perceptive about a depressed mother who keeps visiting the surgery suddenly 'for the children'.

A number of people turn up every year who are either keen to 'have some therapy' without really knowing what they mean, or resigned to the idea that they must, but who are found during the consultation to be so unsuitable for it that it would be a mindless and unconcerned act – both for the patient and the putative therapist – to try to set it up. By 'unsuitable', I mean either that they are so strongly resistant that they would sabotage it at every turn, consciously and unconsciously, or that they show no signs of psychological-mindedness at all – or both. These people are invariably relieved when I say firmly that I am *not* going to refer them for psychotherapy, and that I think it is *not* the right treatment for them. One woman, who was ill, but could only use drugs and psychiatric support, burst into tears of gratitude, and said the decision had made her feel better than she had for weeks.

Another man was so near the edge of paranoid psychosis that it was quite unpleasant being within range of his aura of sarcastic, cold, angry personality; he was seemingly more of a psychopath than I would ever refer for dynamic work. He was a bit late arriving, and seductively held my hand slightly too long on shaking it, calling me by my first name, which I dislike. He gave his story fluently, and I suspect untruthfully; his pale blue eyes held mine unblinkingly, and challengingly, throughout. (I am at a loss to understand where the notion arose that it is desirable and a mark of integrity to look people in the eye for long periods of time; it seems to me unnatural, and discomfort-producing.)

Eventually, I said to this forty-seven-year-old man, when I felt I had got his measure a bit more firmly, 'I don't recall saying that you might call me Nina.' He looked at me sardonically, and said in a humouring sort of way, 'Don't you care for it, then? All right, what would *you* like?' I said coolly, 'Well, I prefer Dr Coltart in this particular situation.' He proceeded to call me Dr Coltart with slight but elaborate emphasis every three or four minutes from then on.

One can't win with such a person, and I imagined the hellish difficulties with counter-transference, which in this case would virtually take the place of transference. I was having problems enough with my own: I had to arrive at some sort of judgement as neutrally as possible about the 'solution' for this character, and I wasn't at all sure I had even located the problem. As it happened, he had said early on that he was here on the advice of a colleague of his, but that he personally didn't think much of the idea; besides, it interfered with a plan he had to go abroad for some years. From the way this was delivered, I imagine he foresaw a pleasurable struggle between us lying ahead, in which I fought for my cause and begged him at least to give it (me) a chance. If this was correct, he must have been disappointed.

Ludicrously, it almost turned inside out. I ended up by strongly supporting his wish to travel – if indeed he had such a thing – and he was arguing, as he thought persuasively, in favour of going into what he called 'analysis'. I explained in some detail what analysis and therapy are, and how they work, and some of the mental characteristics in the patient that make them more appropriate as a prescription. Included in these, I said, was a level of integrity and commitment and seriousness of which I did not think he was capable. His story had been a tangle of changed jobs, abandoned women, and unhappy relationships with parents and brothers, though all slanted in such a way that he seemed to emerge – or rather he intended this effect – always a blameless victim of circumstance. Insight into responsibility for himself and the happenings of his life was markedly missing.

He was injured and outraged by what I said. I seemed to have joined a long trail of people who didn't understand him. I said musingly that I wondered, then, who ever would. He agreed with me pathetically, as if I had offered consolation or spotted a problem. It gradually emerged that his wish to go abroad and take up a job offer in another continent was genuine, and by the end of this interview I was helping him with his plans. I am sure he felt a degree of triumph which enabled him to leave with such equanimity as he had unruffled by me.

Assessment of patients is one area where my medical training has occasionally come in useful, both from the diagnostic and the prescribing angles. Also there is a long tradition in Britain of referral to 'specialists', i.e. doctors with particular corners in the expertise field. As with many things which turn out to be successful, the origins of the consultation practice were almost accidental. When I set up in private practice, I had a number of contacts among psychiatrists in the National Health Service. They were partly baffled, partly pleased at what I was doing. They now had somewhere to send their odd cases, mostly from out-patients, who expressed either an overt wish for psychotherapy – which was just coming into public consciousness in the early 1960s – or who seemed to have the sort of illness which even my most organic ex-colleagues could see might benefit from 'a bit of talking therapy'. Indeed, I would probably have starved rapidly had it not been for this source of referrals; as it was, I was soon looking around for new friends and acquaintances in the therapy world who wanted patients. I had only just begun my own training analysis, so I had only few colleagues in this field; however, once qualified we all needed patients, and gradually my circle of people to whom to make referrals widened.

I will now describe a strange case which frequently made me feel I *ought* to be using my medical skills, and yet which frustrated them absolutely. A young man of twenty came to see me, complaining of losing interest in his work, and feeling as if the world was getting more remote from him. He was undeniably a rather withdrawn and odd person, but he talked fairly freely to me.

He was referred to me by the chaplain of his Oxbridge college, in whom he had confided. The patient came from a landed gentry background, and had had a promising career at his public school, where he was considered well above average, and bore this out by getting a good Oxbridge scholarship. His work went steadily downhill from about his second term, and he became quiet and isolated, which represented a marked change of pattern for him. He felt fed up with himself for his deterioration, and when both his mother and his father wrote to me, it was clear that his superego was largely an expression of parental hopes and voiced expectations, which he was failing.

His father was much more sympathetic, both to him and to the world of psychotherapy, than his mother. A letter from her displayed huge, flamboyant writing, permitting only ten or twelve words to the page. She spoke in barely disguised terms of her total incomprehension both of her son and of what I was or did. Referring to the young man, now twenty-one, deeply confused and wretched, she said, 'he was tired out, but . . . he has slept and eaten a good deal . . . He is at last tackling his thank-you letters and as always is *very appreciative* of his own home. It is a great pleasure to have him home,' (this was well into the spring term when a more appropriate view from her would have been worry that he

was not at college, working) 'and we are all *so happy* together . . .'
There was more in this vein. I talked to his GP, who was very
concerned; he hardly knew the young man, but said the mother
was a terrible woman, domineering and paranoid, 'always taking
against people, the sort of person who will either drive all her
relatives away or end up in a mental hospital'.

Meanwhile, confiding by letter to his chaplain that '. . . there is
no hope, I feel as if I am going to die', the young man came up to
see me for his five visits in just under three weeks. This represented an extended consultation, which I had decided to carry out.
He neither complained of physical symptoms, nor did careful
questioning from me elicit any. He talked freely, with the freedom
of desperation, and said he feared 'dying of leukaemia', and felt he
was 'getting separated from the world'. His GP had arranged for
blood tests to be done, and these showed no abnormality. There
was a slight suggestion of hearing faint voices telling him he was
evil and lazy. The idea of schizophrenia stayed in my mind, but I
had an uneasy, ill-defined feeling this was not right. I was supported in this feeling by some words of Wilfred Bion: '. . . the
divergence between the psychotic and non-psychotic personality,
and in particular the role of projective identification in the psychotic part of the personality as a substitute for regression in the
neurotic personality.'[1] The patient I was so puzzled by was regressed and depressed; projective mechanisms did not seem to
play much part at all in how he operated.

After the fourth visit, I did two things that to this day I feel
relieved at having done, and which, however vague the reasoning
behind them, I think were to do with having had a medical training. I made a comment in his notes: 'There's something odd and
sort of physical about this. He's out of sync with his body as well
as the world. Chemical? What does he mean by his fears of
dying?', and I referred him to a psychiatric, rather organically
orientated consultant, a friend of mine at the Maudsley. On the
fifth visit I discussed this with the patient, and he agreed that we
seemed rather stuck, just as he felt. He went to the Maudsley two
days later. They examined him in every possible way, and found
no physical signs. My colleague nevertheless agreed with the
strange feeling I had had, and continued to see him at weekly
intervals and put him on Largactil, to which he did not respond.
Six weeks later he became quite suddenly ill, and manifested
physical signs of a brain tumour; it was found to be inoperable,
and he died two months after that.

I include this mercifully unique story not because it directly added in any way to my equanimity, but because it taught me something about the value of trusting that whole apparatus, conscious and unconscious, which we bring to our work, and which is called 'intuition', and which in this instance had one of its roots in medical training.

What is intuition? I think there is an ultimately unknowable quality to it, just as there is in every patient, as well as in why and how psychotherapy 'works'. It undoubtedly contains a rich compost of silted-down experience which is daily strengthened, unnoticed, by our work. It could not operate without bare attention, a special kind of detailed scrutiny bound up with a clear mind and with reflection, which I have written about elsewhere.[2] It is of vital importance to learn to trust one's intuition, and this can only come about if one is always on the look-out to test it, and to develop the power to discriminate – itself frequently a semiconscious process – between it and imagination. Only slowly will it become a reliable tool in our kit. It is, however, better to trust it and risk being wrong than to tread too gingerly, which will slow up its often rapid operation, and maybe impede it at source.

The young student discussed above stands out in my mind as probably the most distressing assessment I ever did. He is not a particularly solid example of the value of being medically trained, and yet I am sure that influenced my overall impressions. There have been people over the years, however, whose diagnoses arose almost entirely out of that dimension.

The following vignette contains a warning about the constricting power of a diagnosis. A diagnosis can close the mind, or at the very least limit its scope. It gives us a sense of assurance, of having moved nearer a solution, and indeed, since many forms of treatment depend on it, it is quite desirable that it should – but without suspending thought, or alternatives.

The woman, age forty-five, gave every appearance of being severely depressed. She had slowed down, her affects were blunted, her thought processes were blocked. In this state, she said, with understandable tears, she felt quite unlike her old self, and could not pull herself out of it, no matter how hard she tried. There was enough in her past and recent history to make it seem likely that she had a depressive form of mid-life crisis.

I prepared her for some psychotherapeutic treatment, which was quite a struggle as she was not at all keen, yet showed sufficient awareness of psychological ways of responding and looking at herself to make it a valid plan. I then talked to her GP, who had referred her, on the telephone. It was during this conversation that his mind came free of the sort of bondage I have just described, and he suddenly said, 'You know, I didn't do her thyroid tests. I wonder . . .? I think I must.' It is easy enough to walk through a gate which somebody else holds open. I could see immediately the point of his idea. I refrained from further plans until he had seen her through her blood tests. These revealed a diagnosis of severe myxoedema (inadequate functioning of the thyroid gland); the instatement of treatment was soon under way, and she responded by becoming, very rapidly, her 'old self' again.

Rather oddly, this woman presented a particular difficulty along the way, which I have also re-experienced more than once. She had been quite reluctant to accept a psychiatric referral, and yet after her consultation she was then reluctant to go back to her 'real doctor' to have her thyroid levels assessed. By that time she had pointed herself in the direction of psychotherapy, and was a convert to the idea. I was a disappointment to her; I had not particularly pleased myself either – an accurate organic diagnosis from me would have been much better for my self-esteem. At the same time, I learned the hard way a particular lesson, which has stood me in good stead on at least three occasions since.

Far more difficult, and more common, is a phenomenon which occurs more frequently, namely people who have somatic symptoms, and who are grimly determined that their cause is purely organic, when absolutely no abnormality can be discovered, even on extensive testing. 'Hypochondriasis' is a word loosely used, usually to describe some tiresome, ageing woman. It is in fact a very exact diagnosis of a psychosis. Hypochondriasis is a severe, often monosymptomatic, form of paranoia, and it is such an exact diagnosis that it is a pity that its current fate – becoming a pejorative criticism – has become attached to it. Unfortunately, an equally dismissive and shallow fate has befallen its most likely alternative, 'hysteria'. This, too – at heart a valuable and descriptive diagnosis – has suffered a change of use for the worse, largely because its presentation has changed.

It used to be important to be able to discriminate between hysteria and hypochondriasis; theoretically, in the unlikely event of encountering either, it still is. The aetiology, the presentation, and the treatment are different, as are the affects displayed (if I were to say by the 'sufferer', it would be incorrect). The hallmark of the hysteric is *la belle indifference*, and very striking it was, too, in patients of long ago. The most vivid case I recall was a nun, who was admitted to the Observation Ward of a hospital where I was the house physician, just starting out on the path of psychiatry and beginning to learn how to do assessments. Her right arm (she was right-handed) had become completely paralyzed, and exhibited the classical 'glove anaesthesia', which means she could feel nothing in it over the area which she thought was likely to be damaged, but which does not correspond accurately to the nerve distribution of the hand. These symptoms prove conclusively that hysterical thinking, and false premises, operate powerfully at an unconscious level. Also classical was her smiling, bland acceptance of her trial, as one might think it: she was completely disabled from using her right arm and hand at all, and as she was the valued calligraphic scribe for her whole order, this was inconvenient, to say the least.

We had not yet caught up with the fact that Freud had deliberately stopped using hypnosis for such people sixty years before we still used it, and it was by this rapid means, rather than perhaps months of careful exploratory therapy, that we soon learned about her quite lurid and sadistic masturbation fantasies and her strong temptation to perform the forbidden sexual acts. She was prepared to risk the impatience and annoyance caused to the Sisters and her Mother Superior; after all, she was not to blame. She was being tried by God. Her will was paralyzed below the level of consciousness, and the Sisters could not, in all conscience, be cross with her. In other circumstances, she might have produced the stigmata, had exhibitionism and masochism blended on a different neuronal pathway.

Hypochondriasis is a psychotic illness; and the symptom itself may be madder than a hysterical conversion, which has a distinctly teleological meaning, fairly easily uncovered. The hypochondriac is a paranoiac whose symbolic use of the body is more enigmatic and primitive. Furthermore, the violent projective mechanisms so characteristic of paranoia stay in, or at the surface of, the body; they do not get attached to selected external objects. The origins of true somatic symptomatology are earlier than the development of thought, and, therefore, of speech; this is why they are so hard to translate into language which has resonant meaning for the patient. Hysterical symptoms arise later in the development line, when thought, fantasy, and language are already available. Hence their much greater accessibility to 'translation', and hence the root and stem of the difference between the two psychopathologies.

I have covered the ground here in some detail because I am referring to one of the many diagnostic challenges which arise in the course of doing assessments. Such challenges stretch one's mind, add variety to one's daily practice, and, in their intrinsic clinical interest, contribute strongly to the refreshment and enjoyment of the therapist's life.

Perhaps the greatest challenge in doing assessments and in maintaining the daily practice is to the creative use of experience as time passes. If after thirty years of working, one's style has not changed markedly and deepened, then something was wrong with one's choice of career. This is probably not the case: if one spends a day or so observing how one works now, consciously comparing and contrasting one's technique with what one can recall about the past, most of us would have to acknowledge that enormous evolutionary changes have taken place.

I certainly recall how hampering doubt and anxiety could be, and how much of both there was, and how I longed for greater assurance. Slowly, probably imperceptibly, confidence grows, and eventually we move about in ourselves as we interact with our patients, up and down through the layers of consciousness, following our free associations and counter-transferences in all the directions they suggest; surefooted and aware of the continuing paradox that constant attention, combined with emptying our minds of memory and desire, eventually pay off, and that we have developed our own technique. Consciousness of this, though it is rooted in the unconscious – another paradox – is a source of pleasure and a sense of freedom. It is only after years of working that we realize that not only are we surviving with enjoyment, but we might even be bold enough to tackle a subject of such refinement as the art of psychotherapy.

6
The Art of Assessment

The 'art' of assessment? A bit rarefied? Rather presumptuous? But unless one is so modest that it borders on the pathological, one will be aware of having attained a certain skill, even expertise, in a particular subject close to one's heart. If I were to behave as if this skill has not by now been given so much attention by me that it has been honed into something subtle and specialized, then I would be underplaying my hand.

All therapists do a certain number of assessments, if only with the patients whom they are about to treat in their own practices. There are a great many similarities between the diagnostic consultation, with a view to making a referral for the patient, and a good preliminary interview. Also, a number of therapists are required, from time to time, to carry out one-off assessments.

In previous chapters, through thoughts and memories, and some clinical pictures, the consultation practice has been presented as a fairly straightforward, journeyman's piece of work. To reflect upon these interviews as an ongoing ephemeral art form involves close attention to the apparent trivia, the sorts of subtle minutiae which usually escape notice when the subject of assessment is under review.

Pleasurable as is the whole event, it is the awareness of getting it right, in detail, for each individual, which substantially transforms the assessment interview into a solid plank of the survival-with-enjoyment structure. Each individual imposes minute variations on one's own behaviour, which is both authoritative and intensely receptive. It is the observing and remembering of certain things that seems to transform the meeting from a work-a-day routine interview to the level of art, bringing the most satisfaction to the assessor, and creating lasting memories of hundreds of very different interviews.

I know from long experience that the patient never forgets a consultation. The details of the exchange fade, but a patient always remembers the overall feeling-tone of the meeting, the sense of comfort or discomfort, the colouring, which render it unique in his life. Not only do we frequently prescribe a momentous course of action for the patient's future at the end of the assessment interview, but even as we open the door to that patient we are embarking on an event which will be uniquely memorable for him. We carry the responsibility for meeting the patient face-to-face, as honestly as may be, and working rapidly on all the material we are given, attempting in the process to make it a good memory for him, worthy of its uniqueness.

The assessment that is leading up to referral differs from the preliminary interview of a treatment by oneself. For a potential referrer, it is essential that over the years one builds up an extensive working acquaintance with a large number of therapists of different persuasions. Any committee of which one is a member, any clinical meeting that one attends, offer among other interests an excellent opportunity for getting to know people and filing them away in one's mind for future reference.

It is necessary to maintain this aim consciously in mind at any gathering of psychotherapists. The particular task – an obligation on the regular consultant who is continually adding to her private stores of information – will not be met if one just chats idly to one's neighbour at a meeting; but an interval or coffee break can be used fruitfully to get to know at least half a dozen people, receive a sharp, general impression of each, enquire about their wish for referrals, what kind of therapy they do, and what sort of psychopathology they particularly like to work with.

Correlated with this ever-growing list, it is important to acquaint oneself with the different training organizations, so that one has some clear idea about what the therapist's training is likely to have given him. For my own purposes, I include in the gathering of information a few therapists of entirely different persuasions: I may never, or only rarely, turn to them, but I am acquainted with a few representatives of, for example, cognitive therapy, behaviour therapy, hypnotherapy, acupuncture, bioenergetics, and, most important, good, reliable, middle-of-the-road psychiatry. I am not implying that one will often need to refer patients to these practitioners, though there are occasions when the most sophisticated treatment choice will be behaviour therapy, or good, clinical, medicating psychiatry – even ECT, for which there is still a viable place. From time to time patients turn up who have already received treatment from a member of one of these bodies, and it is as well to be aware of what their experience may have been. One of my most rewarding patients was a Freemason who had fallen into the hands of the scientologists, and only extricated himself with the utmost determination and difficulty.

Through his analysis I learned a great deal about this brain-washing troop of fanatics, which has stood me in good stead on at least three occasions, since there have been other movements during the last two decades whose techniques were not dissimilar.

We now come to the assessment interview itself. From the viewpoint of what one is actually looking for, I consider the backbone of the consultation to be psychological-mindedness. When I was invited to contribute to the *British Journal of Psychiatry*, I listed the nine qualities I think add up to psychological-mindedness, and then discussed them.[1] I will list them again here, briefly, because I believe that assessing their presence – or absence – contributes to the art of the assessment interview:

- An acknowledgement, tacit or explicit, by the patient that he has an unconscious mental life, and that it affects his thought and behaviour.
- The capacity to give a self-aware history, not necessarily in chronological order.
- The capacity to give this history without prompting from the assessor, and with some sense of the patient's emotional relatedness to the events of his own life and their meaning for him.
- The capacity to recall memories, with their appropriate affects.
- Some capacity to take the occasional step back from his own story and to reflect upon it, often with the help of a brief discussion with the assessor.
- Signs of a willingness to take responsibility for himself and his own personal evolution.
- Imagination, as expressed in imagery, metaphors, dreams, identifications with other people, empathy, and so on.
- Some signs of hope and realistic self-esteem. This may be faint, especially if the patient is depressed, but it is nevertheless important.
- The overall impression of the development of the relationship with the assessor.

It should be remembered that it is perfectly possible for a person to come across as being intelligent, sophisticated, capable of sustained thought, aware of symptoms – and yet absolutely not psychologically-minded. There usually is not a strong rapport between the interviewer and such patients, although examples of them are not uncommon, especially in the academic and the general medical worlds. Such people are not good bets for dynamic psychotherapy, though this may contradict their own view of themselves.

For a patient to be deemed suitable for analytical psychotherapy, a minimum of three or four of the above qualities should be present. Patients for whom full analysis is the most appropriate prescription will probably manage all of them; even then the prescription can only be made with confidence if other variables are also present, such as a high degree of motivation which will ensure commitment, sufficient time available, and the ability to pay for it. Very few people turn up for consultation already fully informed about psychoanalysis, and knowing that it is what they are searching for.

These, together with the patients who are more ignorant of our field but who nevertheless turn out to fulfil all the criteria, both psychological and practical, only add up to about five percent of all the assessments I do in a year. The majority of those who are found to be thoroughly psychologically-minded cannot afford either the time or the money for five-times-a-week analysis, and find the idea of three sessions a week more tolerable; they therefore form the majority of the sort of referrals I make from my practice. With very few exceptions psychoanalysts and psychotherapists welcome such referrals, and probably the main bulk of practices will be found to consist of them. Helping the rest of the patients to decide between one and two sessions a week can be a surprisingly tricky task.

There are a small number, of great interest to an assessor with a well-stocked store-cupboard of treatment sources in her mind, who may call for specialized treatment. For example, patients trying to kick an addiction are best referred to a group specializing in a focal technique; a patient with an underlying organic illness may need, before all else, to see a general physician or surgeon – the refinements of this sort of decision-making are part of the art of assessment.

The main contribution to the raising-to-an-art of what is already a skilled craft lies in the combination of knowledgeable, detailed, and ceaseless hard work, and the flowing quality of apparent effortlessness. A consultation on this level would achieve all the practitioner wishes in the way of: past and family history; lucid understanding of what the trouble is; some formulation as to the unconscious aetiology and the meaning of symptoms; a clear directional sense of where, or to whom, to go next; as well as establishing a subtle and deepening rapport with the patient. Such a consultation will serve not only to elicit with clarity much dynamic material, but also is intrinsically supportive, hope-confirming, and reassuring (true reassurance does not require weak, consoling phrases which might be designated 'reassurance' in the everyday sense).

The techniques for this multifaceted piece of work should be tuned to such a pitch that they are invisible. No patient should be aware of the quantity and quality of the skills which are being deployed; no textbook-type language should be used; and the patient's primary awareness of the consultant's state of mind and rapport is that they are relaxed, still, attentive, and concentrated entirely on him.

A minimum of two hours should be put aside for the interview itself, and the consultant will need at the very least another hour later – I suggest within the same day – in which to write a full note, reflect on the referral plan, and to make successful contact with the selected therapist. The process of selection is largely uncon-scious. I find that if I push every bit of data from the interview down into my unconscious 'computer', frequently the name of the right therapist will swim to the surface. I then test it out by conscious reflection.

A deep and thorough assessment cannot be achieved in less than two hours; usually I reserve two and a half because discussion of what is going to happen next may take up to half an hour. It is at that point that the consultant should encourage, and answer, all the questions which arise in the patient's mind when considering his recommended treatment. I think all questions about treatment should be fully and openly answered. One is, as I said earlier, prescribing a momentous commitment – of emotions, time, and money – to a fellow human being, and one has the opportunity to introduce him comfortably to a field which may be strange to him.

This brings me to manners. In the many accounts I hear of assessment interviews, it appears that ordinary good manners are sometimes abandoned at the consulting-room door. The most dis-tressing source of information is the number of patients who fi-nally pluck up the courage to try for a second assessment and referral after a traumatic experience in the first one. There are certain features which turn up over and over again in the patients' accounts of such damaging interviews. While always ready, as one should be, to listen with some scepticism and awareness of distor-tions to a patient's account of a session with a colleague, the repeated weight of the evidence develops an inescapable ring of truth. I shall address some of these through a brief description of what I would advise actually doing. It is the *not* doing of these things which may seem insignificant to the assessor, but which make a marked impression on a vulnerable, anxious patient. It does not seem an unworthy or unprofessional ambition to want to create a good memory in a patient. The consultation is memorable anyway, and the subsequent treatment is likely to proceed with less difficulty if its jumping-off point feels good.

I like to shake hands at the door or in the waiting room, say the patient's name, and introduce myself by name. There is no reason why the patient will clairvoyantly know who you are, especially in a crowded waiting room in an institution; even in your own home you may be mistaken for a receptionist. I accompany the patient to and from the waiting room, and, when I am ready, to the consulting room, indicating where the lavatory is en route (a surprising number of people, who may have travelled a long way or be anxious, or both, want to use the lavatory at some time during the session but are afraid to say so if they do not even know it is there).

In the consulting room I indicate where the patient should sit; a young analyst, reporting on a preliminary interview, once said to me with a laugh, 'She went straight in and sat in *my* chair. Of course, I had to move her.' I did not find this at all funny, and I imagine for the patient it was even less so. It may have been significant, and could have been avoided. I then write down the patient's address, telephone number, age, and check the name of the referrer. Then I lay the pen and paper aside, making it clear that I shall not take any more notes. (I do hope that not taking notes in the presence of the patient is an absolute and unchanging piece of discipline which we share, the only exception I make is for a very intricate family tree, if it seems it may be important.)

While I am on the subject, I want to ask: whatever happened to smiling? An extraordinarily powerful, unspoken myth seems to have steadily grown which says that to smile at a patient is to do something mysteriously awful, not only to him, but to the whole session. I think this is more likely to be about the consultant's perhaps rather precarious sense of her/himself. It seems to me there is something ridiculous, and rather sad, if an ordinary smile, which can do so much to achieve a rapid and all-important relaxation in the patient, is somehow felt to be damaging to the seriousness of the whole event. A welcoming smile at the beginning, and an occasional laugh if humour seems important to the patient –

even more strongly taboo in some quarters – need not betoken an attitude inimical to the assessor's dignity, or that we know the patient is here because he is suffering in some way. Why can't a smile be a small but vital part of the ordinary good manners required by the act of inviting someone to sit down in one's own room to tell one private things about himself?

I open the assessment by saying how long we have got, and that during that time I like to get to know a lot about the patient's life and how it came to the point of his being here now. In the majority of cases this releases the patient into embarking on his story, maybe slowly and hesitantly at first, but there is no need to prompt him further at this stage. All that is required is that one sit still, train one's most concentrated attention on the patient, and start to work.

I want to emphasize here that, first, an assessment is hard work, and second, it should not be organized like an ordinary analytic session. My researches suggest that psychoanalysts are the worst offenders in this latter respect; it is the most common cause of trauma in patients who go away from a consultation in a worse state than they came, and who may be put off any form of therapy for months, years, or forever.

The main body of the interview is the place for some of the hardest work; the stillness in which you sit; the quality of your attention; the constant exercise of memory; the skilful use of brief interventions; the decisions about when, or if, to make a few real interpretations; and the ceaseless alertness to signs of psycho-logical-mindedness are all part of the work.

People vary in their opinions about interpretations during an assessment. For analytical therapists, one or two are essential in order to form an opinion on their reception by the patient. But they should certainly not be all that is said. Furthermore, it is exceedingly important never to arouse, or contribute to, anxiety unless there is still time and opportunity to do some working through with the patient. Yet from patients who have undergone hurtful, counterproductive interviews, I have heard often enough of long silences capped by one or two heavy interpretations dir-ected mainly at the unconscious – which, to an inexperienced patient, is still *very* unconscious – followed by little or nothing more.

I have brought up the matter with some of the colleagues men-tioned: their explanations of the technique, and of the theory un-derpinning it, are so completely different from my own that there is little point in prolonged discussion. The colleagues who operate differently from me will offer the 'stimulus to the patient's anxiety' as a primary reason for making a penetrating, perhaps painful, interpretation. They do not believe it is essential to unravel this anxiety and relieve it before the end of this session: I suppose it is intended to bring the patient more smartly into treatment; or perhaps to give him something to prove that his inner world can be shaken, and to 'work on' in the interim before therapy starts. It may prove to the consultant's satisfaction that the patient can be shaken, and they may feel they have at least got hold of a dynamic theme. But a patient who has stumbled blindly away from such an interview, crying, hurt, and baffled, is exactly the sort of patient who, if he is not too disabled by neurosis, begins to get angry as well, and may well be lost to therapy for a long time. Some of the reports I have heard from patients traumatized by assessment interviews show unmistakable signs of unworked-through sadism directed at a person who is already in a disadvantaged position.

This particular subject makes me want to ask: what about kindness? I do not believe there is anything in our theories which gives us licence to abandon kindness. To be kind does not mean to be sentimental; it is surely one of the many and mixed motivations that drive us to become therapists in the first place.

It is perfectly possible to see something nasty lurking inside every apparently good intention, but this is not the same as saying that goodness is always at heart corrupt. There are good qualities which can more than balance the natural unpleasantness of human nature, which have enormous personal, social, and intrinsic value. Of these, I think kindness is one of the highest goods. It does not need to be expressed directly, either in language or behaviour, but it needs to inform our actions, speech – and therapeutic techniques – rather as a dominant colour can characterize an object. If our aggression is creatively harnessed by kindness, so we can make free use of this powerful combination, it is then possible to be tough, relentless, and confrontative without any fear of hurting a patient beyond the pain that insight brings as it opens up new and hidden views of this personality. Unsmiling, ruthless assaults on a patient are not the only alternatives to the weakness, woolly thinking, and sentimentality of which some people seem to fear kindness must inevitably consist.

After the patient has more or less reached a natural breaking-off point, time for silent reflection should be used by the interviewer. There are subtle body-language signals by which one can convey to the patient that one now requires silence for a while before offering some thoughts and suggestions. Shifting one's position for the first time, looking away and down at the floor come to mind as examples. Eventually I will try to summarize to the patient how his account of his story has led into the problems which have brought him for consultation. Often it is possible to pick up a thread of connectedness and aetiology where none has previously existed in the patient's mind; if some degree of interpretation is needed to make sense of the connection, then it should certainly be made. This attempt at a comprehensible, insightful comment may well lead us into a deeper layer of dynamic, if necessarily brief, discussion.

Time is getting shorter, and the second task of this phase, after the comment as above, is to make one's recommendation about treatment, which again may entail further discussion, and explanation, and, on occasion, some dynamic work on a patch of ambivalent resistance. It is at this last stage of the interview that I think questions should be answered, if possible.

At the end, I accompany the patient to the waiting room to collect his coat, and so on, shake hands and say goodbye, clarifying with him that I will telephone him in a few days when I have established a suitable referral. (Of the reports I have received on traumatizing interviews, five mentioned they were not shown to, or through, the door of the consulting room, and/or that the assessor, having risen to his feet, waited in silence for the patient's departure, without saying goodbye.)

The art of assessment includes having a clear view of exactly what one wants to elicit from the patient during the meeting. I aim for as much of the personal story as possible, short of having to prompt laboriously. I have two main reasons for this. The first brings us back to psychological-mindedness: one is in no position to make a judgement about this unless the patient has talked quite a lot, and therefore, as skilfully and unobtrusively as possible, one wants to enable him to do so. A very silent interviewee may make a very difficult patient in individual treatment, nor is it likely that he will be an active participant in a group. This sort of patient, who almost forces one into a laborious question-and-answer position, may be fairly easy to diagnose, but is difficult to refer, and even makes it hard to know what treatment decision to reach.

My second reason is that a detailed history can be of immense value to the therapist during the course of the treatment. Far less information may be given in ordinary sessions, especially if the patient is ill and preoccupied with symptoms, or is in a disturbed, confused state of mind. All therapy is immeasurably enriched if the therapist has the important relationships of the patient's life clear in his own mind, along with salient points about life events. (Here I am referring to preliminary, or first, sessions with the patient's therapists as much as to an assessment interview; if the therapist prefers to get straight down to treatment, he can ask to read the assessor's notes, and learn some history details that way.)

My feeling about getting a good history is: 'Now's your chance!' It is not good technique, nor often is it possible, to start filling in bits of important data by asking frequent questions once a treatment is under way. Nor do I think it is good technique to rely entirely from the start on the transference, or on you-mean-me interpretations, for information. With no history there can be no delicate nuances of transference interpretation – only abstractions, too generalized to have sharp meaning. In the hands of inexperienced therapists, a clinical seminar based on little or no hard information can be a lamentable event. Unless we expect to be therapeutic by our very presence in the room, and accurately interpretative from some theory-type fantasy of our own, we have to know quite a lot about our patients before we start. Otherwise we are omnipotently practising bad magic. The transference can later be extremely informative, but the point and power of interpretations are enhanced by relating them to the personal life and circumstances of the patient.

As to the question of 'diagnosis', I do not think anyone doing assessment work believes that the conditions we see and treat are properly described as 'illnesses' most of the time, or that they have exact parallels in the physical disorders. For the purposes of recommending dynamic therapy, individual, or group, anything resembling an ordinary 'medical diagnosis' is neither possible nor helpful. The majority of therapists are not doctors, and although I consider it desirable that a primary assessor should be a doctor, the sorts of diagnoses which regular psychiatrists feel the need for are not much use to us.

My reason for thinking that people who do a great many assessments should preferably be doctors is that once in a long while, a disease process which is physical in origin and can be successfully treated as such, masquerades as a psychic disorder; it is infinitely better for the patient if the assessor is able to recognize this. As illustrated earlier the patient may have the dangerous physical illness of decreasing thyroid function, which

may be misleadingly disguised by symptoms suggestive of neurosis or melancholia.

I saw another patient in consultation who turned out to have a
rapidly growing, though fortunately benign, pituitary tumour. It
was as if she was unconsciously far more in touch with her body
than she could, on a conscious level, think about, since she had
developed symptoms of severe anxiety with some depressive colouring. She 'happened to mention' that she had started lactating
slightly – 'Isn't that odd?' In the circumstances it was not odd – it
was diagnostic, and I grasped at this signpost to the right path.

On the other hand, doctors entering our field should forget a
great deal of their medical training as fast as possible. Unless
something physical is really wrong with the patient, the language
and thinking should move away from the medical pattern. Of
course it should be possible by the end of the two hours to say
whether a patient is obsessional, hysterical, character-disordered,
schizoid, psychotic, neurotic, or psychopathic. A narcissistic character disorder, unless extremely blatant, can be almost impossible
to diagnose on first acquaintance, as can a successful false-self
character. I do not, therefore, make much of an attempt at a 'diagnosis'. What *is* important is, first, that we should decide whether
this patient is likely to derive benefit from any of the sorts of
therapy to which we have access; and, second, to put our opinion
into clear, descriptive language. This description may include the
degree of psychological-mindedness; of course one can employ
theoretical language when discussing things with an analytically
trained colleague to substantiate opinion.

On these descriptive summaries, which we reflect on as we
write up the patient's notes later, are based the referrals for
therapy that we make. To fulfil the criteria of the art of assessment, the notes should be full and detailed, and include some of
our own thoughts and associations. If I possibly can I refer the
patient within a week; this is a significant time in his life, and he
will be waiting with eagerness and anxiety for one's telephone call.
It is not good to leave him in limbo for weeks or even months at
this point, and I see no excuse for it. This bit of the job alone may
occupy an hour or more a week. In some ways it can be the most
taxing, and it is certainly part of the art of the whole business.

I do not give patients more than one therapist's name, and I tell
them this at the end of the interview. I will have taken considerable care in placing the patient, first in my mind, and then in what
may be quite a long negotiation with whoever it is, during which I

first establish that she/he has, or soon will have, a vacancy, and then will probably, at her/his request, describe the patient in some detail. If the patient says he wants a list, I ask what criteria he can use for choosing, and we usually then have a discussion on why I am in a better position than he is, at this moment, to select someone for him. This is one of the situations in which I believe that we do the patient no service by assuming a false modesty, and if we cannot use some sort of authority, which derives from trusting our training and experience, then we are playing some game of pseudo-democracy.

Finally, there is the question of payment. Some patients will grumble, or feel outraged, by a high fee; some ask what the charge is when they first telephone or write for an appointment, and that is a good opportunity to be perfectly clear, and, on the majority of occasions, to stick to it. It is only with very rare exceptions that I will reduce my fee, and in thirty years I have only had three or four bad debts. Some patients ask me if they can pay me at the end of the assessment interview; unless there is absolutely nothing more that I am going to be doing I refuse, and say I will send my account when we have satisfactorily established a referral to the person who will be doing the therapy.

I hope I have succeeded in differentiating the art of consultation from the ordinary, everyday, working principles of the task. If the various things I have selected for emphasis seem obvious and uncontroversial, I can believe that at least I have confirmed your own style, with the apparent trivia which may seem insignificant, but which add up to the art of assessment.

7
Stranger than Fiction . . .

A number of people undertake a psychotherapy training quite late in life, after having pursued some other career altogether. I am including this piece of history as support, and as encouragement for a move that can sometimes seem quite drastic, both to the self and to one's circle in the world.

It sounds callous to say that one of the strokes of luck in my life was the coronary thrombosis of a senior colleague; it would be callous if he had died, but fortunately he lived for many more years after this event, which provided a timely bridge for me. I had decided to leave the Health Service when I was a registrar, which was generally regarded by my colleagues as a bold and daring (if they were being polite), or extremely rash and silly (if not), thing to do. But in the larger things of life I have always trusted my intuition, and it has proved a staunch ally in the survival stakes. The trust has always paid off, and from a position of experience I would quite strongly advise that this path is worth following. The change in career, mid-stream, was all part of the sense of vocation, and contributed maximally to my survival-with-enjoyment.

Soon after I had come to the decision to leave the Health Service, one of the consultant psychiatrists at my teaching hospital had a coronary infarction. As well as some sessions at Bart's, he had a flourishing private practice in Wimpole Street, the sort of practice which needs constant tending if it is to continue to succeed. He sent for me, knowing of my recent decision, and asked me if I would act as locum for him until he recovered, which he firmly intended to do. I was delighted at this chance to come to grips with the private sector. It would be valuable experience, and any psychiatric problem faced could not but be good practice for general diagnosis and assessment, which I hoped to establish when on my own.

I worked in the practice three days a week for six months, and during that time managed to get my own private practice sketchily started. Thus I had a real and much-needed bridge, for if it had not been for the Wimpole Street work, I would have had a pretty lean time.

And so started my new life in the world of the psychologically disordered. It would be impossible to construct a hierarchy of the strange cases that came my way, with some completely bizarre person on a single pinnacle at the top, but, first in the Wimpole Street rooms, and later across the years in Hampstead, a number of patients appeared whose stories were to me truly stranger than fiction.

In the Wimpole Street practice, one of the happenings was a weekly ECT clinic. A consultant anaesthetist friend of my colleague would turn up, and – since ECT was far more often prescribed then than it is now – there were always two or three patients from the practice waiting for their treatments; there was a small recovery room where they would rest for a while after the shock had been administered, cared for by the secretary and myself.

The ECT recovery period is not always a peaceful experience. The rarest phenomenon, and the most dreaded by any young psychiatrist, is a 'post-epileptic furore'. In this hair-raising event, the patient, not yet in his right mind, goes completely berserk, charging about breaking things and attacking people; his strength is that of ten. This frightening outburst is heralded by a particular roaring cry which is unmistakable once heard, and gives one twenty seconds to prepare, usually inadequately, for trouble. This frightening event happened once in the sedate rooms of Wimpole Street.

Another vignette particularly stays in my mind. My ill colleague had already seen once an Orthodox Jewish woman who was pregnant. She was in a state of delusional mania, and believed herself to be carrying the Messiah. (Many years later, I realized that this is not an uncommon delusion in strictly religious Orthodox women, at times somewhat alarmingly colluded with by their family. The teaching that the Messiah is yet to come plainly has great potential for influence over the primitive layers of the mind, and after all no Gentiles can safely, or convincingly, lay their hands on their hearts and say that the notion is mistaken.) My colleague was a great believer in prescribing ECT when there was no obvious alternative, which was usually the case in 1960; the major tranquillizers, which, whatever their critics say, produced such a marked change for the better in the psychiatric population, only came on the market that year, and were as yet untried by most of us. My colleague used to say of ECT, 'At least it breaks up the pattern of the thinking', which was certainly true. Whether one could then reassemble the pieces remained to be seen.

The Jewish lady arrived one day, duly prepared for her treatment. The anaesthetist gave her an injection, put a rubber airway between her teeth, and held the oxygen mask in readiness; I applied the electrodes to her temples and administered the shock. To my horror, the top of her head fell off. At least this was what appeared to happen; it took me the longest minute I have ever lived through to realize that as an Orthodox wife her hair was very closely cut, and she was wearing a clever and luxuriant wig. The momentary brief convulsion of the whole body, which is the beginning of the diminished fit that ensues when the shock is given, had jerked her head so violently that the wig had slipped backwards and sideways, giving the unnerving impression that irreparable damage had occurred.

The case which was to be the longest in sheer duration was introduced to me in a way which instantly marked the patient as being more bizarre than one is liable to come across in any work of fiction. Another consultant who occasionally called on my colleague was a general physician specializing in diabetes. He did so on this occasion, and was surprised to see, in his stead, a face which until a few years previously he had been accustomed to seeing among the gaggle of students on a teaching round in his wards. However, he graciously accepted my arrival, and treated my opinion with courteous gravity. As it coincided with his, and consisted of my saying; 'No, I don't know what it is, either', this was not the professional struggle it might have been. He took me to see a well-groomed woman with rich red hair, beautifully clad in an expensive nightdress and jacket, sitting up in bed and staring into space with large, rather mad-looking blue eyes. (This was in a private nursing home which was used for the medically ill, but did not normally admit psychiatric cases.)

The woman had been admitted in insulin coma (not as uncommon then when injected, as rather crude insulin was in frequent use) and had manifested, on examination, not only a low blood sugar, which would be expected, but massive, purulent sores down the fronts of both her lower legs. She was almost entirely mute when retrieved from the coma, so apart from knowing her general history, as she had been a regular attender at his diabetic clinic for about a year, Dr B could not get any further. We both agreed we had never seen anything quite like the oozing, infected areas on her legs. The patient stared past us when asked questions, and did not answer.

As her diabetes had been stabilized, Dr B was anxious to discharge the woman, and with mixed feelings I accepted his decision to take her 'into my care'. She was to go to the Sister who looked after his patients every day, morning and evening, for dressings. It seemed she had no friends or relations, and no next-of-kin was mentioned in her notes, where it was stated that she was a teacher, and Roman Catholic.

I arranged to see her twice a week, not a usual pattern in Wimpole Street, but as she had yet to divulge anything at all about herself, I thought that giving her some space and attention might help. I had just started my own five-times-a-week treatment, so twice did not seem such a lot as it once would have. Also, she gave every appearance of having plenty of money; I was at that point green enough to be concerned about the high level of fees (three guineas a visit!) which patients were required to pay in the private sector.

My patient, who I shall call Miss X, began slowly to answer my more innocuous questions, and I learned she was now fifty, though she looked thirty-five. She had been orphaned at the age of four, when her parents had died in a car crash, and then she had been taken in by the headmistress of a private girls' school in Shropshire, and brought up there in a manner reminiscent of the attic-life of the little rich girl in *The Little Princess*.[1] Miss X had been educated only in so far as her duties as a maid-of-all-work, childminder to the younger girls, and general assistant to the headmistress allowed.

The headmistress, who I will call Miss H, though a powerful and in some ways successful figure, had kept this school running until about a year previously, when, after many admissions to mental hospitals and various suicide attempts, she had finally killed herself with an overdose of barbiturates, which she took regularly in large quantities, and cutting her wrists in the bath. My patient had found her there, eventually, by putting a ladder against the house, climbing up and peering through the window.

Miss X had found herself alone in the world, without proper qualifications, as she said that Miss H had sent her to a teacher training college but had insisted that she return to help run the school shortly before she was due to take her exams. There she had remained ever since, apparently in a state of hypnotic-like dependence on Miss H, in a condition of slavery in which she appeared to have felt quite powerless to alter things.

This extraordinary story took about three weeks to elicit piecemeal, but – as I later realized in the course of my analytic training – during this period, a very dependent, single-minded transference was in the process of finding a final resting-place after a year of hanging loose following Miss H's death. Miss X had drifted to London, hoping for the best. She had kept herself going by picking up supply teaching in schools which were desperate and not fussy about qualifications.

I can only say that the fictional quality of this garishly romantic tale did arouse my suspicions, and I can only add that, having now known this woman for over thirty years, I have found an absolute internal consistency always present in any references to her early life, although the patient did in many other ways turn out to be a pathological liar of quite stunning magnitude. In recent years I have continued to see her once a week, and regarded it as a life-task. I know this patient so well by now, and have survived so much with her, that at times I feel I would do anything to discharge her – and yet I could at no point cast her adrift. She made a go of her life, in some ways better than one might have expected, but it was always with the anchorage of her safe harbour (me) assured. My mind reels to this day when I look back over the various upheavals which occurred in her treatment, let alone in her stories about her life.

But to return to those early weeks, and the mysterious sores on her legs which the nursing-home Sister was dressing every day. The Sister rang me after about a fortnight and said, 'Those sores aren't getting any better, you know. It's almost as if something's preventing them . . .' Almost in concert, the same suspicion entered our minds at the same moment: 'I wonder . . .?' we said, together. 'Could she . . .? How? What with?' I promised Sister I would do my best to find out the truth.

Now, it does not take years of training to recognize that the transference gives power to the therapist, at some times more than at others. I had realized that the bullying, tyrannical ways of Miss H might well have been part of what held Miss X hypnotized in a sadomasochistic prison; that her growing attachment to me was only partly because I was not unkind to her; and I might have to use a bullying tactic to get her to shift psychologically.

At her next session I bided my time until an opportunity presented itself, and the subject of her continued need for dressings came up. I had been silent for a while, but suddenly I said, very sharply, 'You're keeping those things going yourself, aren't you? How are you doing it?' The woman jumped, starting to wring her hands in a particular way I already knew, and stared past me with her mouth firmly shut. I waited and waited. Eventually, I snapped curtly, 'I know you are. You don't want me to stop seeing you, do you? So tell me . . .' I had no intention of abandoning her, but I did resort to the threat.

After about five minutes of wringing and shuddering, and opening and shutting her mouth, the patient at last said, in a faint, gasping whisper, 'Oven cleaner'. I felt the sensation which I believe to be one's hair standing on end. Oven cleaner is almost pure caustic soda in paste form; its containers are heavily printed with warnings about protection for the skin when using it. Sister and I had thought she was simply excoriating the areas. I could only just begin to imagine the blistering pain of actually applying oven cleaner to one's skin, and to an already sore, purulent place at that. 'You mean, that's how you got those sores in the first place?' I asked. 'Yes', she whispered. I asked her why, but this was pushing it too far. Though clever and cunning in some ways, she has never been psychologically-minded or truly introspective, and I think beyond dimly knowing that she *had* to get into care, had to have an authority over her, she really could not say.

This was the beginning of a long, eventful treatment, in which bizarre forms of acting-out such as I have never encountered elsewhere played a considerable part. Sorting out truth from fantasy was a primary and ongoing task; although I said earlier that, crudely speaking, she was a pathological liar, I slowly came to the conclusion that her often pointless 'lies' were more in the nature of fanciful scripts in which she played a dramatic part, and that she would identify with her self-cast roles so strongly that it could not quite accurately be called lying when she spoke of them.

Her early life with Miss H, though no doubt dramatized in the telling, had a solid consistency over many years; this led me to think that the original melodramatic artist was Miss H, and that Miss X's subsequent advanced capacities for romancing and acting-out were the effect of an extensive identification with her and with their bizarre life, rather than that she constructed her stories ('lied') for me. Miss H was admitted to hospital, usually psychiatric, on numerous occasions; so had my patient been, on a lesser scale, and usually for 'unstable diabetic attacks'. Miss H took vast quantities of drugs, mainly barbiturates; my patient only gradually revealed to me that she took Valium in huge quantities, and to obtain them was registered with at least three GPs; Miss H had had a lot of money at some point or appeared to have, and when it disappeared, continued to behave as if she were immensely wealthy; it seemed likely to me that she had been a hysteric, but a manic-depressive one, and that extravagant bouts of spending accompanied her manic phases; she

was eventually declared bankrupt, and was an undischarged bankrupt when she died.

My patient, when I first knew her, appeared to be rich and
extravagant. She went into private psychiatric hospitals, dressed
impeccably, and used to have her hair done, and a manicure, twice
a week – to come and see me. After I cottoned on to this, (which
took about three years, I am sorry to say) I began to go into her
financial affairs in detail, and was stunned by what I found. She
had at least four bank accounts, with huge overdrafts in each; bank
managers seemed to fall for the blue-eyed waif, even as the GPs
did, and I suppose, for a longish time, the various consultants
called in, including myself. She continued to earn a little, from
time to time, teaching in schools, since she managed to evade
questions about her qualifications, or else, I assume, lied. She also
drew unemployment and sickness benefit money, with the collab-
oration of various doctors.

When, eventually I felt I had enough data at my disposal, I
encouraged her to go bankrupt, and steered her through the bank-
ruptcy courts. I realized she could never hope to pay off her vast
debts, and, since she seemed determined to relive much of Miss
H's life, I thought it best to go along with that bit. It was most
instructive, and I have to admit that I quite enjoyed it; especially as
by then – about five years into her psychotherapy – I did feel that
some corners were being turned.

For example, though she never became truthful at all times –
which would have been asking too much of the frail boundaries in
her mind between truth and drama – she did develop a reaction-
formation, over about ten years, to drugs of all sorts, and now
shudders at the thought of taking even an aspirin. She gave up her
pretences of teaching in schools, which always anyway came to
grief; in some mysterious ways I could never quite elucidate, she
either got across other staff and was asked to leave, or she became
phobic about class-room life and left of her own accord. She
continued to coach children with learning difficulties, for which
she had a considerable flair, and she built up quite a little 'practice'
at home by word-of-mouth recommendations, which showed a
reasonably healthy identification with me. I cannot to this day be
sure what sources her income comes from, but since she lives
humbly and quietly in a bedsitting-room, I assume it is not lavish.

When I was bolder, both as a more experienced psychotherapist, and in knowing where I was in the mazes of this patient's
psychopathology, I tackled her diabetes. I realized – again only

after about ten or fifteen years – that I simply did not 'believe' in it. I had been partly conditioned by the seniority of my original colleague, who was looking after her long before all the dramas began to unfold. She still injected herself with insulin twice daily, and would at times, and for years, play her dangerous games of either omitting it or overdosing, and getting a brief hospital admission. I began to think that the whole pattern was an addiction for her, because hers was a curious state in which she behaved 'as if' she were an addict, over this and over tranquillizers, and yet I did not think she was one. I learned to trust a suspicious feeling in me. I told her to stop taking insulin, and to regulate her diet sensibly and not play about with either (this is an example of a kind of bullying in which I trusted the positive aspects of the transference to hold us through its effects). I informed her one-only-now GP that I had done this, and that I supposed she might go into a hyperglycaemic state. She did not. He carried out regular blood-sugar and urine tests, and after a bit of wobbling around, her levels more or less stabilized and have stayed that way for fifteen years. She still keeps to a reasonably low-carbohydrate diet, and tests her own urine at times. There is no doubt that she has a mildly labile blood-sugar, and that this was pumped up into full-blown 'diabetes' when she was casting around for a major and manipulable symptom. She confessed to me only a few years ago that she used to eat sugar lumps and chocolate when she was 'so fed up with Miss H I couldn't bear it another minute'. It was only later she learned to overdose with insulin at times; this also satisfied her dangerous love of risk-taking.

I wondered for years whether *either* she and Miss H developed a lesbian relationship *and/or* she murdered Miss H. I can only say that I think the answer is 'no' in both cases. She is almost unbelievably naïve sexually; I don't think I have ever encountered anyone to whom the whole of human sexuality is such a totally closed book. Miss H, at one point, suddenly came back from a two-month holiday with a baby, which she said she had adopted. But the patient and I have gradually pieced together certain bits of data which say it was, quite clearly, her own (this was a complete revelation to Miss X in the therapy). Its upbringing was almost entirely left to Miss X. And as to murder, I simply do not see her as a murderer. Furthermore, Miss H had made a number of increasingly determined hysterical attempts at suicide, which are always closely described and exactly the same in Miss X's accounts, and, in the nature of things, I think Miss H was heading for success, whether unconsciously or not, I cannot say. Fortunately, this seems to be an identification which Miss X, now a fit, healthy, and slightly demented eighty-year-old, missed out on.

She and I soldier on together, and I suspect there are many therapists who have one or two old lags in their practices, with whom they have had a bumpy and eventful ride for years, but who gradually settle down into a more peaceful evening in their lives, and justify the slow-burning faith which their therapist placed in the process rather than in the patients. One or two friends have said to me occasionally over the years, 'Why on earth don't you get rid of her? Discharge her – go on.' But my answer to this, which some may see as patronizing or soft is, 'No, I can't. You don't throw a dog out on the motorway, just because you're tired of it.'

On the other hand, there are people who are reluctant to come to therapy, though aware that they are in need of it, who stay as short a time as possible, and who tend to depart sooner than we might consider advisable. The limited boundaries of the whole event do not necessarily preclude extraordinary eccentric presentation. Mrs A had enormous, dashing handwriting, in which she wrote in guarded yet garbled terms that her GP had suggested she should come. I also had a very brief letter from him which told me nothing except that she had had psychotherapy before and wanted it again. This lady was seventy-four when I saw her, and the previous therapy had been with a Tavistock doctor, whom she had seen during the war, many years before when the patient was in her forties.

For a start Mrs A looked eccentric. She was a tall, handsome old woman with long, black, Edwardian-type clothes. Her eyesight was poor, which partly explained her huge writing. She lived in quarrelling friction with her old husband, P, who, according to her, was a monster of selfishness. But there was a lot of projection in her account, because his 'selfishness' often seemed to consist of baulking her in her own strong wishes, or not liking things which she insisted on doing because she wanted to. For example, she told me they lived in an enormous, crumbling house with a wild garden, both of which she insisted on looking after herself, as she was somewhat paranoid and did not trust gardeners, cleaning women and the like. One of her husband's 'selfish ways' was not understanding this, and continually urging her to get help in the house and garden, although admittedly it did not seem to occur to him to do anything himself. She either could not or would not drive, I was never quite sure which, so she did all the shopping in her local village either on foot or on a bicycle. A compelling vision was conjured up of this big, dishevelled, wild-haired old woman, pedalling along on an ancient bike, peering short-sightedly through her thick glasses, clutching and balancing plastic bags of shopping. She said that the village children shouted and laughed at her, which was hardly surprising. She must have looked rather like a domestic witch on an earthbound broomstick.

She had multiple, rather non-specific complaints which I supposed added up to depression. She did not sleep well; she had various bodily pains; she could not manage her house; she was angry and fed up with her husband, who insisted on staying in the house, and not moving somewhere smaller; she wanted to cry but was afraid to; she wanted to bang the top of her head; she was preoccupied with thoughts of her parents and how unkind her mother had been to her father; especially in the early hours of the morning she would wake and seethe with rage against her mother who had been dead for over forty years. She was quite sure she wanted treatment, but was very reluctant to have it, as she knew it would be 'so difficult'. Attempts by me to find out what she dreaded so much met with failure. 'I have to do things', she said mysteriously.

We arranged to start the following week, and almost at once she began to write to me, long rambling letters, often two or three between her twice-weekly sessions. These letters were full of appreciation and apologies for her behaviour to me, which hardly warranted so much guilt and shame, and which I therefore thought must be some sort of displacement.

She was certainly difficult to follow at first, and would often tick me off curtly if I did the wrong thing. I had an idea that *she* had a very clear idea about what her treatment needed to consist of, though she found it hard to express. Since there seemed no point in imposing inappropriate therapy on her, I was quite keen to find out more, and accepted her brusque instructions, as well as her dismissiveness, with unforced interest.

She put herself on the couch straight away, and used it in a way I have rarely seen in any other patient. Her behaviour was odd and at first incomprehensible to me. For example, she said she 'needed to make noises' and 'wanted to hurt herself'. She regressed rapidly in each session to a state which I thought was something like a hysterical fugue. She moaned in a low voice which gradually rose to a gasping cry; she twisted her body from side to side and banged her hand and arm on the wall. If I attempted some interpretation, she interrupted me fretfully to say she didn't understand what I was saying, and she wished I'd be quiet. Nevertheless, if I said anything that seemed to hit the mark, she would then cry in a childlike way for some time and say afterwards she felt better. I gradually learned more about the sort of thing she could tolerate, and I spoke rarely and briefly.

When she spoke it was mostly to describe bodily feelings and wishes: 'I feel a pushing on my legs'; 'I want to bang my head'; 'I've got pains in my breasts'; and, with increasing frequency, 'I want to go *down*.' Her movements became more explicit and sexualized. I thought she was enacting a fantasy of some sort of sexual intercourse, and on occasions said so. She snapped rudely that I was not to say things like that; she didn't like it, she had hardly any sex life, her husband had become impotent when they lived in India 'because of amoebic dysentery'. This was a new one on me; and anyway, the 'cause' varied. Some time later she said he'd had an affair and got VD and this had caused the impotence. I was never satisfied that I had been told the real reason for P's impotence, and it occurred to me eventually that it may well have been a chronic depressive response to her own frigid negativity about sex; she sometimes described in disgusted tones how P used to approach her for sex, and how she would reject him.

There was something cold and quite cruel about her. Anyway, Dr M at the Tavistock hadn't said things like that to her, and she didn't like it. As usual, in between sessions her letters apologized both for her 'dreadful embarrassing behaviour', and for her rudeness. I thought that these letters were placatory rather than genuinely penitent.

One day she was clearly enacting giving birth. Though I had on the whole followed her commands not to speak, as it only seemed to waste time, I said so. She replied between 'labour pains' that she only really wanted to 'go down – on my head', and added that the next time she would have to (all this was many years ago, and 'going down' had not arrived in the vernacular with the sexual meaning it has today). Sure enough, in the next session, this large, ungainly woman, her loose white hair tumbling about her face and shoulders, heaved herself up and round on the couch, crawled to the end of it, and dived off. I watched, spellbound. I hardly had time even to be alarmed, though when no sound came from the now invisible figure on the floor, I did wonder whether she was lying there with a broken neck. I sat still and waited; intuition warned me not to leap up and go to her aid. In a few moments she got up quite briskly, sat in the chair while she pinned up some of her unruly hair, and departed saying, 'I feel better. I knew I had to go down.'

At last the mystery became clearer. From then on, she did this diving off the end of the couch about once every three or four sessions. In between she continued the same sexualized behaviour as before, only now she talked more, albeit in a rambling, free-associative way, usually about what she felt in her body, but sometimes about her parents, and especially about her mother's unkindness to her father, and her father's devotion to her; sometimes about the ambivalent relationship to her husband, to whom she was deeply attached in spite of the intense irritation he caused her.

Although she often expressed a wish to 'be hurt', she never did hurt herself. It seemed to me almost miraculous that this heavy, stiff old woman could repeat her ceremonial diving head-first off the couch and never suffer any ill-effects at all. On the contrary, she seemed to recover steadily from her agitated depressive state the more she did it. I decided that her body, in a state of profound and relaxed regression, must become rubbery like that of a bouncing child who picks itself up from tumbles.

Gradually, over the months, I evolved quite an elaborate theory about Mrs A. The first thing which I felt confirmed it, simply from constant attention to the strange combination of what she actually said in conjunction with her bodily behaviour, was that the two were genuinely dissociated. I do believe that consciously she had no idea what her body was saying, and indeed, that if she had, it would have stopped her saying it. I imagined a shocked, horrified response if I were to interpret clearly all, or most, of the theory that I had constructed. Fierce denials greeted even the brief descriptive comments I made from time to time. The almost completely dissociated activity spelled out a fantasy which her conscious super-ego could not have let her acknowledge.

I came to the conclusion that she had a powerfully dramatic Oedipal fantasy of a sexual relationship with her father which resulted in a pregnancy and the birth of a baby; but that at a certain point in the fantasy she became the baby and it was essential to get herself born. I realized it was important to her to control her own birth. Several pieces of history came out which contributed to this idea, including the fact that her mother was said to have had a late miscarriage when Mrs A was four. She had no memory of this event; in fact, her conscious recall was fragmented, and did not in any case extend much beyond the age of seven.

I thought it was just possible that her father had abused her sexually in some way, and that this was a memory retained only in her body. I treated Mrs A about eighteen years ago, and the advances in understanding of incest as described in recent literature had not yet begun. The idea seemed vaguely preposterous then, in the light of the patient's family history, and especially the father's upright, Christian, regular-army personality.

Nevertheless, it seemed to me to contribute to the understanding of some of the things she said, and some of her fixed emotions; for example, her fanatical loyalty and devotion to her father, which was always spoken of in the context of her mother's cruelty and disdain towards him (which I came to think was partly her own projections) – and often also towards her, Mrs A (because she required punishment for her Oedipal triumph); and again, as I have indicated, the amount of guilt and shame she constantly expressed to me over things that she had done – consciously, she meant – in my presence (which did not justify the guilt and shame she felt); and, finally, her scornful (phobic) reaction to sex as an adult alongside her intense and knowledgeable involvement in it in her fantasy life.

The idea of her father and her having a sexual relationship would not seem so alien to us today, but I doubt if even now I would broach it with Mrs A. Her massive denials made it difficult even to interpret to her 'something you might have imagined, or had a sort of daydream about', as I occasionally phrased it to her. This was after I had suggested to her one day that she 'had a fantasy about giving birth', which seemed obvious enough. 'Don't use that word!' she shouted. 'I can't bear you saying "fantasy". I told Dr M the same thing. I don't have that sort of thing. I never did. We never wanted any children. And anyway, I told you, I never liked sex, and P was impotent most of the time.' It seemed to me that the magnitude of her conscious repudiation of sexuality was in direct inverse ratio to her unconscious preoccupation with it. But psychologically-minded she was *not*, and she developed no insight worth the name.

There was something about the very fact of coming and making use of the therapeutic container so dramatically which did seem positively beneficial to her. She said herself that, in spite of the shame and embarrassment, she couldn't have gone through 'it all' on her own, and it had become imperative to do so. She acknowledged before a year was out that she was much better, and began to miss sessions. The domestic and marital difficulties of which she had complained so bitterly seemed to fade away. She and P had an enjoyable holiday in their motor caravan driving through France. In truth they were a game old couple who liked adventures, and her accounts of past holidays of this sort unwittingly showed P in a much better light than she normally granted him. This trip signalled the end of her therapy, rather to my surprise. She never formally terminated with me; she wrote, cancelling a couple of sessions after the holiday, then a couple more; she made special reference to the complicated, long journey she had to undertake to reach me (the first stage on her bicycle); this had not been felt to be an obstacle when her need was great, but now, in her improved state, it seemed almost unbearably difficult. Then she said she was anyway so much better that she didn't think she needed any further appointments. These were not just brief notes – they were long, expressive letters about her current well-being, their journey through France, and her life in general. She wrote at increasingly long intervals for a few months, and then her letters ceased.

I occasionally wondered what bcame of her. She and her husband were old, and getting older and more vulnerable. They were pretty well alone in the world, as they had no relatives, and neither was friendly or sociable. I wondered particularly whether she could possibly remain psychologically well, since I did not think anything in her strange hysterical personality had really changed. I assumed that she had literally had a 'breakdown', from which she then recovered. For me she was one of the most odd and absorbing experiences I ever had in the consulting room; an experience, I thought, in which I had seen and learned a great deal, and yet had done practically nothing. I relished the extraordinary contribution she made to my store of vivid memories. The years went by, and I heard no more of her. What a contrast to the other patient I described, Miss X, whom I could not, and still cannot, dislodge. So different from each other in many ways, and yet so similar in respect of their stranger-than-fiction selves.

It feels to me important for several reasons to include in this exploration of surviving-with-enjoyment as a psychotherapist some of the more unusual of my clinical stories. One reason – perhaps the strongest – is my wish to highlight the extraordinary constancy of the intrinsic interest our work offers us. I can think of very few other jobs which provide such a high and reliable level of absorbing fascination, surprise, challenge to our skills, and stimulus to fresh angles on life. Then there is the paradox that neither can I think of many jobs where the practitioner is so firmly enclosed within such a rigid, specialized, and unchanging form. Day after day, for the whole of her working life, a psychotherapist with a full private practice sits still in exactly the same chair, in the same room, seeing a relatively small number of the same patients – what a recipe for boredom and dullness this repetitive discipline could be! And what saves us from this boredom? The infinite changes rung on the details of the characters and their material, which, hour in and hour out, appear in the therapeutic space of the consulting room, demanding endlessly varied mutations in our involvement, thinking, speaking, decision making – the possibilities themselves, while subtle, are indeed infinite.

Finally, I know from long experience that listening to, or reading, a case history is always welcome. I said earlier that I knew I wanted to be a psychotherapist because I so enjoyed listening to people's stories; whatever the mixed reasons for it, I am pretty sure this characteristic is widely shared by my psychotherapy colleagues. These are the stories of patients whom I have seen and treated. If I am right about the unceasing intrinsic interest, not only of our own work but also of other people's, then I hope that these examples of clinical stories, which add a certain quality of pleasure to the process of survival, may be specifically enjoyed by you all.

8
Leisure and Living

So far, I have approached this survey of life as a full-time working psychotherapist from various angles that converge on the practice itself – training, building the practice, clinical work, consultations, and assessment – all subjects which arise from my own experiences of our common tasks. In this last chapter I shall be more directly autobiographical. The writings of analytical therapists are on the whole deliberately impersonal. A tradition has evolved whereby – except in predictable ways, such as a clinical presentation – one omits self-reference. This feature has developed almost a quality of taboo, and to my mind our literature is sometimes the poorer for it. Where better to go against the received style and reveal something more of oneself than on the subject of personal ways of being?

Being a full-time therapist is a sedentary job. It is probably the most sedentary job there is, because we learn to sit peculiarly still. There is little opportunity for getting up and walking about, as other sitters-down-to work do about every half-hour. We cannot shuffle and fidget, nor, by the time our technique has strengthened and we have practised close free-associative attention for a year or two, do we really need or want to. We cannot spring up and check what we are about to say or do in a textbook; by the time we think of saying it, it is too late, and is probably arising from the unconscious anyway.

The analysts of the early generation, especially those who came to England with or at the same time as Professor Freud, used to knit during sessions. Anna Freud was one of those, and I can call to mind at least six others – including one man – who knitted. I find this almost impossible to imagine; even if they were such perfect knitters that there was no question of stitch-dropping, it cannot be an entirely unconscious activity, and the patient must have been aware, at the very least, of tiny sounds – clickings, friction of arm and hand movements – that the analyst was dealing in to the patient's session time.

Because therapists need to sit still for many hours of every working day, it is especially important that they plan ways to provide the necessary contrasts for themselves. It is likely that in the basic, physical sense, taking a modicum of exercise may help one to survive. One has only to dig and mulch two square yards of a flowerbed after sitting in the therapist's chair for eight hours to develop that sense of freedom of movement, alertness in one's very perceptions as well as one's muscles – a kind of glow, which it is so easy to mistake for moral achievement. I use this example because, much as I believe that having and working in a garden could be one of the strongest factors assisting survival in a therapist, I myself have only achieved this since partial retirement. This does not devalue gardening in the here and now, but it makes me realize more acutely what I already knew through the years: that in an ideal world, all psychotherapists would have a garden.

Simply making the sedentary body do some work for a change has short- as well as long-term benefits. Not 'going for a walk' – which has always seemed to me especially boring and pointless unless the walk is a real hike, in lovely country – but a game, such as squash, is excellent. It demands a huge deployment of energy, and steams off all the suppressed aggression of our daily work, in which aggression usually has to be channelled into sublimated form. Swimming, too, more than repays the inevitable tiresomeness of getting to the water, undressing, drying, and dressing again; it uses all one's muscles, and as a bonus offers a primitive sort of satisfaction in the embracing, supportive qualities of the water itself.

But perhaps even more than the body, the spirit, in a job as absorbing and demanding as ours, needs stimulation, change, refreshment, expansion. What is important is that we understand this from our earliest days, and set about it actively; I would not consider, for example, that slumping in a different chair in front of a television has much to offer. Having said that, the diversions we choose will cover a wide range of enjoyable sources of psychic nourishment, my only stipulation being that they should *not* be concerned with analysis or therapy. For my own refreshment I read modern novels, listen to music, and, whenever I can, look at paintings. Degrees of effort involved in these probably widely shared diversions add a sharp tang of enjoyment to their pursuit.

Which brings me to travelling, the most obvious and elaborate contrast to the sitting-still life of the therapist.

There is something daunting about the notion of travel; also evocative. Huge words like 'travel' produce a great cloud of images; a mix of passing snapshots of all sorts of places one has actually been to, snatches of flights and train journeys, and a ragbag of forgotten scenes and maybe bits of fantasy. The very idea of travelling throws the switch of fantasy, and among these jigsaw pieces are images which have an ancient feeling to them. For example, I can locate a feeling of rushing along very fast in a kind of enclosed carriage or cart, which I remember from at least the age of five; perhaps it has its root and stem right back in my mother's womb? Certainly in a pram.

I began to travel quite soon after the war, when the journey was often adventurous, and there were poverty and hardship to be conquered if one was going to get abroad at all. In 1947 I managed to get to Switzerland for five months by grafting myself on to a diploma course at the University of Lausanne; this was supposed to be a fruitful way of using the time before I went up to Somerville to read French and Spanish. Actually, it was a front, but for something equally fruitful. I had no intention of taking the diploma, and only went in to the University three or four times. But it was a way of getting out of deprived and rationed England to the truly unimaginable wonders of Switzerland. In the immediate post-war time of stringency, I had no qualms about taking this grant, nor have I to this day. That time was memorable and a good start to adult life.

The art and the secret of successful travel is xenophilia. I am not referring here to a love of foreign places, though of course that is almost a given. I refer to a very special form of it, which is making friends with foreigners. Youth is the time for making friends, and friendships are one of the strongest staples for happy survival. In retrospect, as far as I can tell it was purely a chain of happenstance that produced a number of friends for me over the years, who eventually came to the end of whatever it was that had brought them to England in the first place, and returned to their own countries.

In 1950, when I came down from Oxford and before I went to medical school, I travelled for six months in the United States with an American friend who had been reading PPE on a Fulbright Scholarship. America was virtually a closed door to my generation at that time, indeed to most people over here, as we were prohibited by government decree from buying any dollars at all. But this friend had stayed at my home during vacations, and ultimately returned my hospitality with magnificent interest in her own country, where she had a large number of geographically well-situated relations and friends from having moved about with her father, who was a US Army Colonel.

The wonder and excitement aroused by the luxuries of Switzerland were multiplied almost to an infinite degree by the great treasure-house of the United States. In 1950, bread, butter, meat, bacon, sugar, eggs, chocolate, and petrol were still tightly rationed in England. War-time children in Britain were in fact very healthy on the narrowly restricted, almost vegetarian, diet that we were obliged to eat; but it meant that one of the most striking contrasts in the States, in evidence the moment one stepped ashore from the boat, was the food. I have visited the States several times since then, recently to give seminars and papers, when I am generally professional and grown-up; but delightful as all these trips have been, none compares in exquisite specialness with that first time, over forty years ago.

Other friendships, too, turned into passports. I worked at Claybury Hospital, a big psychiatric asylum in Essex, for three years. There I got to know a New Zealand doctor, who finished her analytic training and went home to become the only psycho-analyst in New Zealand. It is entirely thanks to her not only that my seven visits to New Zealand have been some of the best travelling of my life, but that I am writing this at all. Dr Denis Martin, one of the great pioneers of the therapeutic community movement, who sadly died much too young, had recently set in train a whole lot of changes designed to turn Claybury into a therapeutic community, and succeeded, more or less. As one of his innovations, he had started a weekly group for the resident doctors, which included the New Zealander and me. She and I fell to talking one day, and she told me she was doing the analytic training. 'What's that?' I asked. She told me, adding, 'Why don't you do it? I think you'd enjoy it.' So I did.

This simple story is not far from the exact truth. I have frequently been surprised at just how many people come into the analytic world after years of familiarity with it – extensive reading in the right texts, perhaps an analysis already under their belts. I, however, was absolutely, deeply ignorant. I suppose I must have heard of Freud, because people at my level of gross over-education usually had. But I certainly hadn't read any, and didn't even know that psychoanalysis happened in England, let alone what it was; or that Freud had come to live here, or anything about him. I do not think I have ever come across anyone in the British Psychoanalytical Society who embarked on it all in quite such a lamentable state of ignorance. I imagine I was accepted for the training because I was such a *tabula rasa* they felt they could imprint me with anything.

What the New Zealand doctor described had a valency which was waiting to find its exact matching molecule; I recognized the 'vocation' when it came to find me – I went out to meet it with a strong confidence that this was It for me; and it was. I had by then discovered psychotherapy, and it more or less fitted my life's ambition, which was to listen to people telling me their stories. A certain element of psychopathology, induced by a fracture in my own story, contributed to the vocational sense, as it so often does, of deep interest in the life patterns of others, especially as, in tracing the pathology in them, my own reparative drives could come into play.

It has been a great bonus that several of my foreign friends were interested in their own countries and prepared to travel about in them, often in their own cars, with a visitor from abroad. It is entirely thanks to this happy combination that I have been all over New Zealand, Israel, and large stretches of both Australia, and the United States.

Travelling in a country where not only the language, but even the script, is inaccessible, can be unnerving, especially now that the days of simply shouting English rather slowly seem to be past. Although some of my most refreshing and rewarding journeys have been in the company of different friends, I have also travelled extensively on my own, and the sensation of being totally incapable either of speaking or of reading any street-signs, maps, newspapers, or notices can be challengingly eerie. This has not occurred often, but the odd occasions are memorable for the experience of a kind of impotent helplessness which is not quite like anything else. The challenge is exciting, and there is also a particular sort of enjoyment in the experience I would not have missed.

There is, however, a quite different type of aloneness, in which one can feel as solitary as in a Bangkok market, yet be surrounded by hospitable, well-wishing strangers. You, the survivor, are unchanged; it is the milieu, and the reason for being in it, that have radically altered. I refer to travelling to another country in order to lecture or give seminars. This may not come everybody's way, and that it came mine I ascribe largely to a matter of luck and one momentary inspiration.

My bit of luck was the moment of inspiration which made me give the title 'Slouching Towards Bethlehem' to my first paper. Had I been more experienced at giving papers, I might not even have allowed it headroom. (It was at an English-speaking conference in 1981 entitled 'Beyond Words', a subject which, I note with interest, cropped up again in 1992.) There is something that seems to stick in people's minds about the title of my paper; it has turned out to be memorable, a piece of luck quite unanticipated by me. I have often thought gleefully to myself since then, when suddenly appreciating that I am in Washington or New York or Sydney or Melbourne, that if it weren't for long-forgotten 'Slouching Towards Bethlehem' in people's preconscious, I probably wouldn't be there at all.

My three lecturing and teaching trips to the United States and one to Australia have all been in the last decade. Such trips, in spite of being worked very hard, are wholly enjoyable, and an excellent injection to one's self-esteem. One could, I imagine, feel quite lonely, as, surrounded by pleasant new acquaintances, one is nevertheless fundamentally alone, in one's hotel room, and between working periods. This suits me admirably, and I find the whole thing a refreshing change (i.e. it has survival value) from everyday work in the practice. The opportunity to see new places, landscapes, art galleries, and so on is immense, and then there is the bonus of new ideas, new faces, new acquaintances – perhaps even new friends.

It is not difficult to get onto one of the 'circuits', and I would advise shy younger psychotherapists not to hang back and think self-deprecatingly that it could never happen to them. I suggest picking a subject one is interested in, writing a paper about it, and letting it be known around and about that one is willing to talk about it – and perhaps about other things, too. This takes a modicum of self-confidence, but it does not have to be pushy or noisy. We can have little idea over here how grateful many therapists are to see a new face with a few different ideas in its head.

Also, most foreign societies inviting practitioners from Britain are both more well endowed and more generous than the British, and less hung-up about discussing money in the first place. From the point of view of our welcome, we have to remind ourselves that in Australia there are, for example, only twelve members, and, when I was there in 1989, one student in the Adelaide Psychoanalytical Society; and only one psychoanalyst, Gregorio Kohon, in Brisbane, with a handful of Australian-trained psychotherapists and psychologists. The hunger for new ideas, or just new angles, on dynamic therapy is extreme. In the United States, although psychotherapists are by no means isolated, they are, or seem to be, quite delightfully pleased to see visitors from Britain who may bring a new slant to the old stuff. They are also generous with funds. So don't be too retiring about your skills; deploy them as and where you can, and you will find that your survival is the stronger for it.

Finally, on the subject of getting out and about, off the beaten tracks of our practices and the numerous lectures, conferences, and meetings which are all connected with psychotherapy, I would include the maintaining of good contacts with one's family; and – for therapists who have no children – especially with those members of the family who do have children. Friends, of course, can offer the same kind of enjoyment. I do not mean that there is a great deal of emotional gain from visiting aged great-uncles or distant cousins; but a good, solid relationship with a sister or a brother, which will, by definition, cover virtually the whole of one's life with all its stores of shared memories, can occupy a most pleasurable place in one's world.

For me there is something very satisfying in being an aunt: one has none of the worries and responsibilities of parenthood, which the post-war years seem to have multiplied for all who venture into family life; and one has all the fun of being a special figure to them, with the opportunity for close relationships with each of them as they grow up.

Godchildren can produce similar gratification, and several of my friends have provided them, managing to overlook the fact that in my case the title is by courtesy only, and not likely to produce spiritual value for the children. The value for the god-parent attaching to the special relationship can be delightful and rewarding, and I have enjoyed these various children to the full for many years. I think it is legitimate to have included them here, for it is not just the body which cries out for a change of activity in our sedentary lives, but the mind and the spirit also. We do ourselves and our patients no favours by immersing ourselves in psychotherapy from morning until night forever. Unless we want to become distortedly narrow in our outlook and thinking, we urgently need the nurture of change – if we are childless, the instructive, enriching influences of children in our lives can be one of the most refreshing experiences.

Something that has cropped up many times is a particular reaction to the news that I frequently travel alone, and show every sign of greatly enjoying it. This links up with a much larger subject – being alone – and for me represents a choice.

The reaction to which I refer is one of astonishment, and often a kind of anxiety. People who react like this in turn astonish me, though I should be accustomed to it by now. They often question me closely as to whether I shall be 'frightened' of travelling alone, and how I set about it. Often, too, I get the impression they do not quite believe me when I say it is extremely enjoyable in all sorts of ways; such people tend to think I am making the best of a bad job. This is not the case, but I do not press the point. They are convinced of their view, since they are unable to identify imaginatively with mine, and I do not care to sound defensive or as if protesting too much.

The larger question, which I find more interesting but which perhaps is harder to ask, is about the whole life choice of being alone. The choice of independence, the struggles to find out and practise what I had meant, early on, by this strong but hazy concept, has been a deliberate one.

Long before I became the therapist whose means to survival we are reviewing, I followed the intuition which told me that, for me, being alone was the route to survival-with-enjoyment. I stress that this is *my* choice because it is a minority view. Nevertheless, I am aware that in the world of psychotherapists such individuals exist. In the 1970s I noticed with surprise that what felt like a conscious preoccupation had been unconsciously influenced and supported by what was happening in the world around me, especially for women. What I am speaking of here is a lifestyle, or journey, which, as it has turned out, is virtually peculiar to women; it is women therapists – who are nowadays in a considerable majority – who will more instantly recognize news from one of their number far along a peculiarly twentieth-century feminine journey. This is not to say that some men do not also choose the solitary path; they do, but they are fewer in number than women.

The personal inclination towards a life which is fundamentally solitary must have many and varied origins; I think the emphasis on solitude rather than just 'independence' is unusual. As it happens, I know a number of people in the same position, apart from the therapists mentioned, but I think this is a natural consequence of recognizing certain qualities in kindred spirits.

It is an *ongoing* choice, one that is made early on in one's adult life, in the stages of youth when choices about lifestyle are most naturally made, and when the various alternatives are more freely available. One finds oneself, however, re-making the choice in numerous different contexts as the years go by. Travelling I have referred to already. There are a number of others, either about living day in and day out, or about doing things that simply crop up in life. I don't mean going out to dinner or having someone to stay for a few days, but more time-consuming and committed happenings: working on a long project, sharing living space with another person, and, of course, 'having a relationship' – and how one slowly learns to recognize that the choice of a largely solitary lifestyle need not debar one from the fulfilment of an apparently conflicting need for love and relatedness.

It is important to be clear that I am talking about *choice*. There are a lot of people who live alone and do not like it and have not chosen it; those of us who have are on the contrary deeply content with the choice, which is sometimes clear to people without too much explanation.

A recurring difficulty is that of strong pressure, from a number of directions, to change the state of independence. Pressure to change may come both from within oneself and from without; that from within has to be worked through, and this is where the sense of clear choice stands one in good stead. It took quite a lot of analysis, self-analysis, and ordinary psychic hard work for me to learn thoroughly that I was, and am still, called upon to defend this way of life.

The reasons that I can easily express, and which are most easily received, are that I need a lot of time alone to digest and reflect on my work. A dynamic therapist lives with a high level of psychic pressure, and I find I need peace and silence not offered by the consulting room in order to maintain the wellsprings of my own psychological refreshment. There are, of course, many psycho-therapists who are able to combine successfully having a family with maintaining at least a part-time practice.

Psychoanalytical therapy tends to protect those few who, like myself, are not natural joiners, and who do not derive enjoyment and support from being part of an association which offers the company of the like-minded. For many people, however, joining one or more of many organizations is a widespread and acceptable way by which they obtain support, friendships, and pastimes. Whatever the interest – be it popular or esoteric – there is sure to be a society that is built on sharing it.

One automatically becomes a member of one's training society upon qualification as a therapist. There is no strong pressure to attend all the many and varied meetings which the organization convenes, as there are always plenty of colleagues who want to. This is what I mean by 'protection': one is obliged to join, but once a member, obligations are not heavy. However, if you are grateful to psychoanalysis for what you have received from it, you may wish to put something back by working for your own and/or also one or more of the various analytical psychotherapy associations. Analytical therapists, and especially psychoanalysts, also seem to be inordinately fond of giving food and drink parties – largely for each other – and, as the Solitary does not take pleasure in such events, I have avoided them. I have, however, worked on one or other of the training or administrative committees for the last twenty five years. In retrospect, my ten years as director of the London Clinic of Psychoanalysis stand out as having been the most challenging, absorbing, and consistently enjoyable, and many excellent memories of it survive, as do friendships with my Directorate members.

It is only from within an organization, particularly one with a highly specialized focal interest, that one begins to perceive one of the main features which make me sustain a more isolationist position, which, for me, has such survival value. Although it probably varies greatly in degree, there is a defensive quality about many of these organizations that encourages a natural human tendency to split and project the 'bad' outside the group in an attempt to manage ambivalence that may be hard to contain constructively within it. Almost by definition groups form themselves into hierarchies, both inside and outside, relative to other groups, and rivalry develops. Unfortunately, if the association or society contains two or more distinct groupings, perhaps based on radical, but contained, differences of opinion over theory and its application, then an uneasy, paranoid atmosphere can appear within the boundaries of one overall organization.

It is sad to have to come to terms with the fact that this phenomenon is quite startlingly true of the psychoanalytic and analytic therapy associations. In describing the training required to become a therapist, I indicated earlier that the sooner a reduction in idealization of psychoanalysis – and its practitioners – begins, the better. But on qualification, one may still have a strong tendency to idealize psychoanalysis. At the very least there is a hope that the intensity with which the subject matter – the human personality – is studied will encourage the greatest possible use of insight as a moral function, especially in the continuing development of the self. There is, however, still a wish to find that analytical therapists will be – should be, somehow – good human beings, or better than most people.

I do not think this is just a wild, childish fantasy, although knowing a lot about how the mind works does not seem to render us more subtle or strong on the moral plane. The British psycho-analyst Neville Symington was bold enough to say he often thought the net result of a full, exhaustive analysis was to weaken the ego, and increase the vulnerability and dynamic importance of the narcissism of the individual.[1] After prolonged observation, I can only agree.

I deeply believe – and by now have many years' experience to support the belief – that to cultivate not only faith in what we are doing, but also a working philosophy of life that is not based in psychoanalysis, militates against the undesirable analytic effects as summarized by Symington. Since I wrote 'Slouching Towards Bethlehem' faith has been a recurring theme of mine.[2] Not, how-ever, with a capital 'F', which refers to the Christian Faith, in my conditioned mind at least. It is as well to clarify this point because it will not coincide with everyone's view of where the 'F' is, if indeed it means anything to people at all.

Our faith as therapists, that what we are doing is eminently worth doing, day by day, 'without memory and without desire', is only one of its manifestations. Yet it may well be our most pre-cious possession, for without it I fear we would often be lost in confusion, not-knowing, or despair in our long, drawn-out rela-tionships with people who are unhappy, and who put a truly awesome trust – faith – in us to help them through their dark nights of the soul.

If we are going to contribute to our own healthy, happy survival as therapists, we need to cultivate two parallel faiths in our work. When people deliver themselves trustingly into our hands as their therapists, unless they know a considerable amount about psycho-therapy, which many of them do not, this means exactly what it says: they put their faith in *us*, as people. It is only experience which enables us to feel their faith is justified. At the beginning of a career as a therapist, faith in ourselves will of necessity only stem from trusting our wish and intention to do well by these people and to become good therapists; all we have is our awareness of a vocational sense, a strong motivation, and the experience of our own therapy – including an identification with the self-confidence of our own analyst or therapist – on which to rely. When faced with our patients, aware of our inexperience and ignorance, a quantum of anxiety is realistic. It is then that a parallel faith in the therapeutic process we have been trained to use holds us, and evolves quite rapidly with practice – probably more rapidly at first than our faith in ourselves. Until we begin to trust our slowly growing skills, faith in ourselves is tenuous, and sustained largely by patience and hope. Finally, perhaps ten years on from qualification, we realize that faith in the therapeutic process has kept us going until faith in ourselves has drawn level; then the two blend, as anxiety fades and un-self-conscious relaxation becomes the keynote of our daily work.

Some of us feel the need to develop a moral philosophy or even a religious discipline alongside the practice of psychotherapy, especially if we are to avoid the trap of investing psychoanalysis with philosophical or religious significance – a mistake Freud took care to warn against.[3]

When there was relatively little analytic literature around, the writings of Freud were read by those who were interested – and not only practitioners – rather as instalments of Dickens's novels used to be eagerly awaited in the late nineteenth century. It is probable that Freud's distinctive atheism had a considerable impact on a British culture which, apart from that of the Jewish population, was far more permeated eighty years ago by Christianity than it is today. Recently, when I started re-reading Freud from a particular angle, I gained the impression that he couldn't leave religion alone. It even occurs to me that he may well have had a primitive form of religious temperament, one of its signs being a fascination with religion, an inability just to take it or leave it. The to-and-fro movement, rather like Freud's description of the cotton-reel game (now you see it, now you don't) is scattered periodically through his writing. Religion certainly annoyed Freud, which is significant in itself when one considers how much attack and polemic he avoided and rose above, simply saying, 'Never apologize, never explain'.

The trouble with psychoanalysis is that it is such a massive subject, and so completely devoted to the exacting study of the most absorbing thing in the world – ourselves – that it offers scope for many interpretations, including the religious. Some of the signs of investing psychoanalysis with religious significance include devotion to the point of fanaticism; exclusive absorption; the ascribing of omnipotence to certain individuals, or techniques; and the implicit belief in the ability to possess the truth. These are all attitudes which belong more properly in religious categories. As I think that in a paradoxical way this is a degradation and distortion of the power of psychoanalysis in its own sphere, I will move on to the logical alternative: the therapist's need for a philosophy of life that is *not* psychoanalysis, which can provide a vital ingredient in survival.

The promotion of the 'good' – honesty, integrity, sensitivity, and so on – and the reduction of the 'bad' – lying, cheating, stealing, self-absorption at the expense of others – which therapy inevitably entails are also the substance of religious and philosophical systems the world over. The difference is that the motive for practising psychotherapy is not to exert moral pressure, but to heal. To try to perfect skills that enable us not only to work on our own development, but also to assist others to achieve clearer, less self-deceiving minds and to take more responsibility for themselves, is a way of being that is 'good', and falls into the moral order.

The universal existence of religions suggests that human beings have never found it easy to be 'good' just by the light of nature, and are considerably helped by adopting a system, and trying to live within its teaching and discipline. This is as much the case today as ever it was, and there is nothing about psychoanalysis which meets this need, or exonerates us from the common struggle with moral problems, or makes their day-to-day solution easier for us.

I believe that people generally seek and welcome some authority over them which, to use some of the primary language of psychoanalysis, offers assistance in the normal human struggles of the ego against the self-willed instinctual impulses of the id, the harsh criticisms of the superego, and the demands of the external world. There are many who need to feel devotion to a figure, either divine or charismatic, within that system, even a longing to depend on an authority, perhaps to be loved and cared for in return for obedience and submission.

In this need for a powerful figure we can see the bare bones of the invention of God. It is to such needs that we can ascribe the power of the great monotheistic religions – Judaism, Islam, and Christianity. Echoes of this need also appear in a powerful secular system like psychoanalysis. All the organizations based on it, however democratically constituted, throw up outstanding charismatic figures, around whom different schools of thought – often as near to doctrines as makes no matter – group themselves, and who are remembered after their deaths with an unambivalent devotion approaching reverence.

It must be hard for an analytical therapist to believe in God; I would imagine that a certain amount of mental gymnastics must occur, arranging for a few lacunae and elisions. There are, nevertheless, some therapists who quite clearly achieve this, and are satisfied with whatever formulations they have arrived at or accepted. I know of several in London, though of these the majority are mystically orientated Jews, inclined towards the Hassidic tradition; in the United States, there is a minor tradition of Christian believers within the practising psychoanalytic fold.

Long ago I heard the expression 'a God-shaped gap', and I was very taken with it. I did not stop being a Christian because the atheistic Freud and his teachings made me see a different light. I had already been through a process which in religious circles is known as 'losing one's faith'. It happened quite suddenly, but obviously a lot of preparation and reflective inner movement preceded the experience. It is an experience which vividly illustrates the difference between Faith as employed in a theocentric religion, and faith in the therapeutic process and in ourselves. One cannot suddenly 'lose' the latter irretrievably as can happen with Faith in God or supernatural doctrine. One can have periods when it is at a low ebb, or suddenly confirmed, or shaken by depression and anxiety; but it has a solid, tried-out, earthy quality, and no leaps in the dark are necessary to sustain it. However, someone brought up in a Faith and practising it well into adulthood hinges a great part of her moral development and life philosophy on it, and does not want to lose all that as well. These are by then very integrated, and in my case continued to be so through my analysis, but without the sustaining matrix of Faith itself. These seven years were in some ways, spiritually speaking, a time in the wilderness; what they told me clearly was that psychoanalysis was no substitute for a good working religion.

The analysis was extremely interesting, and I valued it as a professional technique I felt thoroughly at home with. It also gave me the opportunity to repair the traumatized aspects of my psyche, and I still regard it as a powerful factor contributing to healthy, long-term survival. I imagine there are many therapists who feel the same way. We are all obliged to undertake a personal therapy as a fundamental feature of our training, and a significant number of future therapists – often gifted, disturbed people – welcome the opportunity to have a good treatment 'undercover', so to speak. I would guess that any student who does not use their therapy as thoroughly as possible is less likely to survive with a growing sense of freedom, enjoyment, and creativity. Regret for lost opportunity, and pain arising from unhealed areas could get in the way of the self-forgetfulness which is ultimately so desirable.

For me, much of the interest of the personal analysis was connected with the study of what my newly lost religious Faith had consisted. It certainly reinforced the bulwarks against any nostalgic or sentimental temptations to return to the fold. I came to see clearly a natural human tendency, observable in babies from the earliest days, to split 'good' and 'bad' into 'me' and 'not-me'. What is intolerable or forbidden or difficult for the self has to go somewhere; this, combined with the conditioned longing for care and nurture – ultimately for union with the most intensely desired sublime Other – is a recipe for a powerful, dependable, authoritative God. In the religious context, much of the 'bad' goes out into the world, and some stays in the self, but is mitigated and forgiven by the 'good', which is largely projected into God. Put like that, the essentially primitive infrastructure of Faith is more clearly revealed.

What I valued in my own therapy was the gradual increase in understanding of the sources of religious faith which led to a greater sense of informed responsibility for the self. This was one of the features which psychoanalysis shared with Buddhism, and which made Buddhism (the only a-theistic religious system) so readily appealing to me when I came across it.

I began to suspect that the best substitute for God-directed prayer – an important ingredient for an active Christian – was meditation. Any set-up which taught meditation became a sign-posted area for investigation. An intensive weekend meditation course I attended was run by a Theravadin Buddhist monk who was one of only four Western monks, trained in Thailand, in this country. I was lucky: it is as important to have a good meditation teacher as to have a congenial, well-trained personal therapist. From him I learned the basic principles of the two main forms of Buddhist meditation, 'observing the breathing' and 'watching thoughts', which take one towards pure concentration, and I practice them to this day.

It would be difficult to assess how great a part this practice has contributed to my survival-with-enjoyment. I am in no doubt that it, and the ongoing effects of the analytic therapy, merged to provide a strong foundation for the living out of the rest of my life. The strength of this blend is immeasurable in its value to me. I have never been aware of dissonance, only of the continuously potentiating effect of the one – psychoanalysis – on the other – Buddhism – and vice versa.

The Buddha was not a god. There was nothing supernatural about him. His teaching was entirely the fruits of his own years of reflection on the workings of his own mind. The Buddha was an astute psychologist, and I do not think I am stretching a point when I say that some of the written-down transcriptions of the Buddha's oral teachings remind me of such papers of Freud that blend clinical and theoretical material. The Buddha was fond of personalized stories ('clinical vignettes'), and, allowing for some archaism in the translated language, and for a more consciously moral stand than Freud would have allowed himself, there is considerable similarity.

Both the Buddha and Freud were brilliant teachers: simple, clear language; grasping the attention of the audience; plenty of clinical illustration; no avoidance of sharpness and criticism where they felt it was warranted; and the constant aim of increasing our psychological understanding – are all factors common to both. Free-associative introspection – for dynamic therapists during a session, for Buddhists in meditation – leads to a deeper and more subtle knowledge of one's self and emotions, and of how self-deceptive we can be through our psychic defence systems; insight is the goal, and, based on new insights, changes in behaviour. Analytic changes occur less consciously than in Buddhist practice; nevertheless, they are more actively represented. The Buddhist aim is mainly to let go of conditioned responses, especially those of greed, grasping, and holding on. Psychoanalysis and Buddhism are the only systems that make sense of the undoubted psychological fact that we hold on to habits and ways of thinking which are actively unpleasant; both help us to develop the skill to let go of such painful and irrational behaviour.

There is nothing particularly comfortable about Buddhism, which is tough and austere, but it is eminently satisfying. One of its most attractive aspects is that there is no more stress on guilt than on any other conditioned emotion. Guilt is fundamental to Judaism and Christianity, and therefore strongly permeates Western culture and psychological development. All therapists, whatever their orientation, know that guilt, both conscious and unconscious, is at the heart of much Western psychopathology. A considerable amount of therapeutic ingenuity is devoted to disentangling and eliminating neurotic guilt, itself consequent upon deviations from super-ego prescription. Elimination of guilt through insight is often not enough to achieve peace of mind; drives to reparation and expiation often have to be satisfied in compensation for the preceding or not fully resolved guilt-feelings.

In Buddhist psychology, since guilt is only one of many transient emotions, all of which are entirely dependent on habit and conditioning – none has more or less weight than any other – there is far less masochistic addiction to self-blame, dramatic breast-beating, and *mea-culpa* attitudes. Although at first quite difficult to become accustomed to, this can be one of the most marked sources of relief to the Western mind. In place of the massive psychic structures occupied by neurotic guilt and its sequelae, in Buddhist psychology there is a section of the teaching which speaks not of 'sins', or sources of guilt, but of what are called 'hindrances'. These, which include rage, envy, greed, laziness and doubt, are presented not primarily as 'bad', or as things to feel guilty about, but as sources of suffering, and things which, if tackled properly with insight, can lead to resolution of what Freud called 'neurotic misery'.

The heart of the whole practice is formal meditation, designed to clear the mind and open it to self-knowing, truth, and understanding; worrying and constant thinking are laid aside, and a kind of empty, alert stillness is aimed for. This provides the best condition in which insight may flourish and be skilfully put to work; the undesirable and unnecessary nature of much that we have either grimly endured, or even cherished as an essential part of our own character, is more easily seen, and such things can then be let go of, increasing our inner detachment, peace of mind, and freedom from subtle forms of suffering. And faith sustains the whole process; faith, as in psychoanalysis, that the process *works*.

My aim has been to indicate our need for faith. Neither Buddhism nor psychotherapy require Faith in the sense of credulity. The New Testament says, 'Faith is the substance of things hoped for, the evidence of things not seen.'[4] Here, St Paul is referring to the kind of irrational faith that requires a leap in the dark. It can only be faith with a capital 'F'. We are told to have faith in something which we have no real evidence for, and we cannot expect any. The Buddha often said, 'Don't just take my word for it; try it for yourselves.' He appealed to pragmatic sense and to experience. He was not enjoining faith with a capital 'F', but faith based on our own personal testing of the process described in his teaching.

I am not attempting a doctrinal exposition, or a sermon, or a promotional puff for something that has been so important in my own survival. What I hope to pur across is an idea of the compatibility of Buddhism with psychoanalytic therapy. As therapists, and as Buddhists, we are not required to make moral judgements, only psychological ones; we sit quietly, often in silence, in a way that is often like meditation, with people whom we are endeavouring to help to get to know themselves in more creative ways, in order to reduce their suffering, which is rooted in misdirected attachments, and also reduce the hindrances which add to their misery.[5]

Patients require to make sense of what we say, and we *should* make sense. However intuitive our logic, and native intuition is to be encouraged, we should be able to work out with a patient the logic of what they are doing to produce their own unnecessary suffering; insight is not going to function without understanding. We need to have faith in the slow, complex, intricate processes that we set in train, but we do not need either our patients or ourselves to have unreasoning faith in us as if we were God.

As therapists we lead such isolated, peculiar lives – alone with a few people who become temporarily extremely dependent on us – that it is fatally easy to slide into a state of omniscience and omnipotence, two of the greatest occupational dangers of the job. Only constant, appraising attention to our own technique, and respect for the patient and the process, will save us. Buddhist practice also needs faith; it only 'works' slowly, and as a result of unremitting attention. It is the very same faith as that required for the practice of psychotherapy.

I have, I hope, demonstrated that faith in our own choices about how to live out our lives, whether in the depths of our work or in the refreshing spaces between our practice hours, makes for freedom and enjoyment, and thus contributes constantly to healthy survival-with-enjoyment.

Notes

1. SURVIVAL-WITH-ENJOYMENT
1. S. Freud, 'Analysis terminable and interminable' in Standard Edition vol. XXIII. London: Hogarth Press 1937, pp. 216–53.

2. PSYCHOANALYSIS vs PSYCHOTHERAPY
1. See N. Coltart, 'Analysis of an Elderly Patient', *International Journal of Psychoanalysis* vol. 72, part 2 (1991), pp. 209–19.
2. See N. Coltart, 'The Assessment of Psychological-mindedness in the Diagnostic Interview', *British Journal of Psychiatry* vol. 153 (1988), pp. 819–20.
3. W. Bion, *Attention and Interpretation*. London: Tavistock Publications 1970, p. 73.
4. N. Coltart, 'The Silent Patient', *Psychoanalytical Dialogues* vol. I, no. 3 (New Jersey 1991), pp. 279–93.

3. APPARENT TRIVIA
1. C. Bollas, *Forces of Destiny: Psychoanalysis and Human Idiom*. London: Free Association Books 1992, pp. 77–92.

5. THE PLEASURES OF ASSESSMENT
1. W. Bion, *Second Thoughts*. New York: Jason Aronson 1967, pp. 43–65.
2. N. Coltart, 'Attention', *British Journal of Psychotherapy* vol. 7, no. 2 (1990), pp. 164–74.

6. THE ART OF ASSESSMENT
1. N. Coltart, 'The Assessment of Psychological-mindedness in the Diagnostic Interview'.

7. STRANGER THAN FICTION . . .
1. Frances Hodgson Burnett, *The Little Princess*. London: Penguin 1984.

8. LEISURE AND LIVING
1. N. Symington, *Bulletin of the British Psychoanalytical Society*. Privately published, 1990.
2. N. Coltart, 'Slouching towards Bethlehem', in G. Kohon, ed., *The British School of Psychoanalysis*. London: Free Association Books 1985, pp. 185–200.

3. See N. Coltart, 'Is Psychoanalysis Another Religion?', in I. Ward, ed., *Essays*. London: Freud Museum 1993.
4. Saint Paul's *Letter to the Hebrews*, chapter 11, verse 1.
5. See W. Rahula, *What the Buddha Taught*. London: Faber and Faber 1982.

Further reading

Note: references to Freud's works are to the Standard Edition, translated by James Strachey and published in London by the Hogarth Press.

Alvarez, A., *The Savage God*. London: Weidenfeld and Nicolson 1971.
Balint, M., *The Basic Fault*. London: Tavistock Publications 1968.
Berke, J., *The Tyranny of Malice*. New York: Knopf 1989.
Bollas, C., *The Shadow of the Object: Psychoanalysis of the Unthought Known*. London: Free Association Books 1987.
Coltart, N., *Slouching Towards Bethlehem and Further Psychoanalytic Explorations*. London: Free Association Books 1992. (This collection contains all the author's writings quoted in the text, except for Chapter 2, note 2 (also Chapter 6, note 1) and Chapter 8, note 3.)
Freud, S., 'Formulations on the two principles of mental functioning'. 1911. S.E. vol. XII, p. 218–26.
Freud, S., 'Recommendations to physicians practising psychoanalysis'. 1912. S.E. vol. XII, pp. 111–20.
Freud, S., 'On beginning the treatment'. 1913. S.E. vol. XII, pp. 123–44.
Freud, S., 'Observations on transference-love'. 1914. S.E. vol. XII, pp. 159–71.
Freud, S., 'Remembering, repeating and working-through'. 1914. S.E. vol. XII, pp. 145–56.
Freud, S., 'Mourning and melancholia'. 1917. S.E. vol. XIV, pp. 237–58.
Freud, S., 'The Ego and the Id'. 1923. S.E. vol. XIX, pp. 12–59.
Freud, S., 'The Future of an Illusion'. 1927. S.E. vol. XXI, pp. 5–56.
Freud, S., 'Civilization and its Discontents'. 1930. S.E. vol. XXI, pp. 57–146.
Ferenczi, S., *Clinical Diary*. Cambridge, MA: Harvard University Press 1988.
Greenson, R., *Technique and Practice of Psychoanalysis*. London: Hogarth Press 1981.
Haynal, A., *The Technique at Issue*. London: Karnac Books 1988.
Humphrey, C., *The Buddhist Way of Life*. London: Allen and Unwin 1969.
McDougall, J., *Plea for a Measure of Abnormality*. New York: International Universities Press 1980.
Needleman, J., *On the Way to Self-Knowledge*. New York: Knopf 1976.
Nyanaponika Thera, *The Heart of Buddhist Meditation*. London: Century Hutchinson 1962.
Scharff, D., *Refinding the Object and Reclaiming the Self*. Northvale, NJ: Jason Aronson 1992.

Symington, N., 'The analyst's act of freedom as agent of therapeutic change'. *International Journal of Psychoanalysis* vol. 10 (1983), pp. 283–91.

Symington, N., *The Analytic Experience*. London: Free Association Books 1986.

Winnicott, D.W., 'Hate in the counter-transference' in *Collected Papers: Through Paediatrics to Psychoanalysis*. London: Tavistock Publications 1947.

Winnicott, D.W., *The Maturational Object and Facilitating Environment*. London: Hogarth Press 1965.

Zetzel, E., 'The so-called "good hysteric" ' *International Journal of Psychoanalysis*, vol. 49 (1968), pp. 256–60.

Zetzel, E., *The Capacity for Emotional Growth*. London: Hogarth Press 1970.

| *Index*

16310902R00072

Printed in Great Britain
by Amazon